A COMPLETE GUIDE TO SEXUAL INFECTIONS

ALSO BY STEPHANI COOK

Second Life

Healthy Sex

. . . And Keeping It That Way

by RICHARD LUMIERE, M.D., and STEPHANI COOK

SIMON AND SCHUSTER • NEW YORK

Color drawings follow page 144.

SIMON AND SCHUSTER and colophon are registered trademarks of
Simon & Schuster
Manufactured in the United States of America

10 9 8 7 6 5 4 3 2 1
Pbk. 10 9 8 7 6 5 4 3 2 1

Library of Congress Catalog Card No.: 83-60640

ISBN 0-671-45493-5
      0-671-45899-X Pbk

This book is dedicated to John B. Springer

The information in this book should help you to educate yourself so that you are a more responsible—and healthy—sexual partner . . . and a better-informed patient should you develop an infection. It is accurate to the best of our knowledge and consistent with the research available to us at the time of writing.

Information does change, however, and *each individual is different, so please be aware that this book is intended only as an introduction and guide to the subject of sexual infections and in no way should be considered a substitute for the attention of your own doctor or medical facility.*

The authors wish to thank

Priscilla Schaffer, Ph.D., Director of Tumor Virus Genetics at the Sidney Farber Cancer Institute and Professor of Microbiology and Molecular Genetics at the Harvard Medical School

and

Richard J. O'Reilly, M.D., Chief of Bone Marrow Transplantation and Attending Physician in the Department of Pediatrics at Memorial Hospital at Memorial Sloan-Kettering Cancer Center, Lila Acheson Wallace Professor of Pediatric Research at Memorial Sloan-Kettering Cancer Center and at Cornell University Medical College, Associate Professor of Pediatrics at Cornell University Medical College, and Associate Attending Pediatrician at the New York Hospital

for their help in the preparation of certain parts of this manuscript.

Thanks also to John O'Grady, M.D., and Armando Grassi, M.D., for their advice and suggestions.

CONTENTS

PART I

PART II. THE INFECTIONS

PART III. YOUR SEXUAL HEALTH

PART I

EVERYTHING YOU NEVER WANTED TO KNOW ABOUT SEX

or WHY SOMEONE NICE LIKE YOU WOULD WANT A BOOK LIKE THIS

We're all nice. And clean. And careful. And if that were worth a whole lot in the sexually active climate of the 1980s, there would be many fewer sexually transmitted diseases around, and a lot less misunderstanding and paranoia about sexual infections in general. Because anybody can get a sexual infection. And many of us will, at one time or another, if we lead sexually active lives.

If you have never caught anything, you're lucky. (There are over *ten million* new cases of venereal disease every year.) It is also possible that you *have* caught a couple of things you didn't recognize, or that "went away" . . . or that there was no name for (the famous "nonspecific"). Public attitudes toward sexual infections are much like those of the ordinary person: the less we know about this, the better we are all going to feel. There has been inadequate funding for research, insufficient record-keeping, and a consignment of the concerns of the sexually active to the armed forces and inner-city VD clinics.

The reality is that every one of us who is sexually active—even if it is with only one partner—is at some risk for sexual infection (not *all* sexual infections are even "caught"; a few can "develop" through factors other than recent transmission), and many of us will be exposed to disease-producing organisms somewhere in the course of our sexual lives.

So this book is not to scare you or dismay you. It is to share important information that every sexually active person needs. To be forewarned—and fore-educated—is to be forearmed; the first line of defense *must* be adequate knowledge, and **being a responsible adult** (even if you are still in your teens—one in seven teenagers has a sexual infection) **means being informed and prepared.**

Almost all of the infections we discuss *can* be cured—if you know what to look for, what the danger signals are, and what to do. The real problems come from those infections that are missed, or are *not* attended to. The better acquainted you are with some of the occasional (and usually minor, albeit upsetting) complications of the pleasure of sexual freedom, the less likely they are to get in your way, to confuse and panic you, and to cause anxiety. Or make you sick.

Nobody ever caught a sexual infection from reading about it, and knowing something about such infections does not somehow render you more vulnerable to them.

It is what you *don't* know that can hurt you.

How Come Sexual Infections Have Gotten More Common Than a Cold?

Everybody's scared. The sexual battlefield has always been mined . . . but now there are many more troops on it, and the view from the trenches is depressing. Is everyone really at greater risk? Or are we just noticing the problem more?

It's some of both. More people are unquestionably doing more things with more other people: no one would dispute the observation that there has been a significant shift in sexual mores and practices in the last couple of decades, and where there is more frequent and varied contact, there is likely to be more passing of infection. At the same time, although there has been an absolute rise in the number of *reported* sexual infections, societal bias *against* report and recognition of this considerable public health problem seems to have been transformed into a bias *for* such report and recognition: what used to be ignored, deflected, or hushed up is appearing on prime-time TV and the covers of national magazines. In short, the perceived epidemic of sexual infections is partly real, and partly a reflection of reporting bias and bandwagonism.

Apparent rise in the incidence of sexual infections is owing to, among other things:

- People are finally ready to see sexual infections as a health problem that is "classless." *Anybody* can get a sexual infection, and the people for whom this *is* news are resoundingly middle-class.
- Middle-class health problems are rewarded with attention from the (predominantly middle-class) health establishment, leading to a rise in medical interest and research in identifying and isolating pathogens, and in diagnosis and treatment of the infections for which they are responsible. (A considerable side benefit of this attention is the increasing sophistication about the *complications* of sexual infections, especially those that are asymptomatic. The infectious origin and cause of many cases of sterility—particularly in women—and the effect of some infections on the fetus and newborn are only two examples of the potential long-range impact of an untreated sexual infection.)
- When a health problem becomes mainstream, it is attended by all the trappings of other mainstream health concerns: scrutiny in the media, attention from high school counselors and college health services, and the broadening of the experience of the medical generalist (the good old family doctor or the avuncular gynecologist) to include venereal conditions s/he never saw or treated before.
- "Raised consciousness" mitigates the stigma (although perhaps not much) of "having something": **people who *suspect* a problem are not only better prepared to recognize it, but are more likely to seek treatment rather than to hope it "goes away."** Hence, higher consciousness encourages a higher report rate, which results in higher numbers.

On the other hand, *actual* increase in the incidence of sexual infections is probably owing to:

- A dramatic rise in the average number of sexual contacts per person: more people *are* involved with more other people, with the increased risk of exposure to disease. And sexual practices have become more varied, inviting infections to turn up in relatively unexpected places and forms. (The crossover of herpes simplex infections is only one example: Type I used to be confined to the mouth, and Type II to the genitals. The crossover rate is about 20% currently, and rising.)

- Ours is the first generation to abandon barrier methods of contraception (the condom, diaphragm, and spermicidal foam and jelly). Barrier contraceptives have the added advantage of being at least partial barriers to the transmission of infection.
- Furthermore, the IUD—and, in some cases, the Pill—makes a woman more rather than less susceptible to a sexual infection, the IUD because the cord hanging into the vagina is a sort of highway for infection, and both the Pill and the IUD because of changes in body chemistry. (New research on the Pill, however, indicates that it may also *protect* a woman against some infections because it maintains a mucus plug in the os of the cervix—the entrance to the uterus.)

More sexual infections? Probably, but we are certainly not going to hell in a handbasket because of the sexual revolution. More awareness? Definitely. And it is all to the good. To everyone's good, because **the more we know, and the more alert we are, the better we will be at protecting ourselves and others.**

SEXUAL ETIQUETTE

or SO THIS IS WHY THEY CALL IT A SOCIAL DISEASE

There is one thing about sexual infections: You get almost all of them from other people, usually in the most intimate circumstances possible. (The difference between these infections and other communicable diseases, then, is merely where and how you get them, rather than that you get them at all.)

Most of the trauma of sexual infection is psychological and emotional rather than physical. Indeed, we would not be nearly so upset by someone's announcement that we had been exposed to a cold; neither would we be afraid to seek treatment for something curable because of shame, only to find ourselves later with very serious complications because of our reticence. Sexual infections, in that sense, certainly *are* social diseases, because their seriousness is often in direct proportion to the social and psychological problems we have with them and the consequent unwillingness to deal with them. (Herpes is only the most extreme example of this syndrome.) "Social" is an important modifier of the concept of "disease."

One of the most difficult situations any of us will ever find ourselves in is the sharing of the unhappy news that we have either "got something" or have exposed someone else—someone whose caring and respect we probably seek and/or count on—to that "something."

None of this is easy for either party, because whether the "something" is as common, minor, and simple to eradicate as crabs, or as potentially serious as syphilis, or as incurable (currently) as herpes, the trauma of loading that unpleasant information onto someone else—or of having it loaded onto you—is much the same . . . and most of us will share identical feelings of self-loathing, anxiety, and the sense that we have been punished for the pleasures of our sexuality. Some people break up with those with whom they have shared an infection through sheer shame; others break up with the person who has exposed them to something with contempt for their "dirty" partner—which is often contempt for oneself, or misdirected anger, for the "sin" of allowing oneself to have that sexual relationship to begin with. (The concepts of "right" and "wrong" grind into operation distressingly fast when relationships go over such a bump. Or even when self-image alone is jolted.) It is not unusual, furthermore, for people who have had a run-in with a sexual infection to have arousal problems for a while afterward, or even to decide to be celibate—either as atonement, or simply to protect themselves (although they are frequently protecting themselves less from another infection than from feeling uncomfortable about being sexually active).

All these reactions are natural and understandable, given the fact that our sexual psyches have yet to catch up with our sexual behavior. Where a gap like this exists between what we do and what we are willing to accept about ourselves, guilt and anger and anxiety almost always creep in, along with a kind of "magical thinking."

Of course sex is healthy: pleasurable, and good for you too . . . if you go into it with a healthy body and a responsible and healthy attitude. But when something goes awry, most of us "open" people draw blanks on how best to handle the situation. For the *teller* there are questions of what to tell, how to tell it, and to whom. For the *tellee*—the one on the receiving end of the not-so-glad tidings—the question is one of response. Whichever you are, it is good to remember not only that it is frequently hard to know where an infection originally came from (which means that the teller is not necessarily the source, nor the tellee the offended party), but that you are probably somewhere in the middle of a chain of infection no matter what, and that you have responsibilities—no matter what your role—to everyone else in the chain.

FOR THE TELLER

There are some communicational strategies that can help you in floating down a bomb like this—rather than dropping it with explosive results—without in any way compromising your responsibility to your partner(s). **It is important to keep in mind that the issue of "guilt" is less significant than the issue of *responsibility:* because so many of these infections can be asymptomatic, the buck stops with the person who has the symptoms.** You owe it to yourself—and to everyone you are aware of in a chain of sexual contacts—to *tell each person . . .* as you would want to be told. Who knows where it came from? The important thing is for *all* of you to get rid of it.

How to Tell

This is probably not the time when being brutally direct will earn high marks. When you talk to someone—either in person or over the phone—it is considerate to make sure that s/he is in a situation in which s/he can ask necessary questions and give vent to anxieties. A little lead-in like "Are you alone? There's something we need to talk about" warns the person that if s/he is giving a dinner party, or is having a business meeting, there is something to be communicated that needs his/her full attention. It is cruel to tell a person only enough to make him/her anxious and upset without the opportunity to question you closely because it is an awkward moment. If you are pressed, you can warn the tellee further by saying something to suggest the intimate nature of the conversation, such as "This is very personal. Do you want to call me back at a time when we can talk?" By this time most people begin to get the drift. At least this allows the tellee a little control when s/he may feel that s/he has lost it.

You can introduce the particulars by saying, "I just got back from my doctor, and you should know that I have had a positive test for such-and-such." Saying it this way—even if you are mad as hell—implies blame no more than it accepts it, and allows both of you to take a deep breath and talk about the situation like adults. After all, these things do happen.

If You Know Where You Got It and Have to Tell Someone Farther Down the Chain

It might help matters to add an abject apology, saying you know where you got it and reassuring your tellee that it wasn't him/her, and to offer to pay any doctor's bill. Be prepared to say what kind of test you had, how long you have had your problem, what to expect, and—as far as you know—the chances of your friend's having been also infected. Expect anyone who is told that s/he has been exposed to a sexual infection to be both angry and bewildered. Try not to get defensive. *Understand what your friend is going through.*

If You Know Where You Got It and Have to Tell the Giver

It is hard, when you are in this position, not to start screaming and throwing things, or at least being accusatory. For argument's sake, let's assume—as you might do—that the giver didn't *know* that s/he was infected: in this case, you are doing him/her a big favor, and your tellee should be grateful rather than angry or defensive, particularly if you are not on the attack. If in the course of a conversation you get the sense that what you are saying is not news to the tellee, you can't be faulted for letting it rip . . . while reminding yourself that it's not a great character recommendation, and what were you *doing* with this person in the first place—or worse, why weren't you informed as soon as s/he found out?

Either way, *a tellee who is known to be the giver can almost always be counted on to be defensive.* Try to remember that the *two* of you (or maybe more) have a problem that needs to be attended to, and that you will not gain anything by doing more damage than has already been done . . . even in righteous anger.

If You Don't Know Where You Got It and Must Inform All Your Contacts

Couch what you have to say in the knowledge that *you* will be considered the culprit simply because you are the bearer of bad news, that people will be angry, and that *you* will get defensive. Again, *understand the reaction of your tellee(s). Be generous. Be calm.*

There is nothing wrong with saying that you don't know where you got your infection; the person you are speaking to may be the one with the silent case. Explain this. And to make things easier both on yourself and any tellee(s), it doesn't hurt to imply that your possible sources of infection are very limited indeed; even if your calling list looks like a modest version of VD Central, you don't need to add to the anxiety of this particular tellee by suggesting that there are legions of sexual contacts involved.

It is nice to insert a note of identification and concern. After all, *you* were taken by surprise, too, and it is no pleasure to have to call in the first place: "I'm terribly upset about this, but I would never forgive myself if I hadn't let you know. And please, let me know what the doctor says." This last can be important to you in figuring out where the problem came from, and where it might be going.

FOR THE TELLEE

As unpleasant as it is to be notified that you "may have something," remember that it is no picnic for the teller to let *you* know . . . and further, unless you are reassured otherwise, *you yourself may be suspect.* You are also going to have to remember who your other contacts are, if any, and let *them* know, so it's important to get the details—and get them right—without either being defensive or coming apart in rage.

If the Teller Seems to Think It Was You

Keep the teller calm, and try to get the whole story. What does s/he have? What were the symptoms, and when did they appear? Has a doctor been consulted? (You would be surprised how many people will make that accusatory call before an itch or a discharge has even been diagnosed.) Ask yourself as honestly as possible whether you might have had similar symptoms and dismissed them, or, if you noticed something, when it was. **Remember that not having symptoms doesn't mean not having an infection,** so the retort "Well, it wasn't *me*—I haven't noticed anything" is unproductive. It is better to question the teller closely on why s/he thinks it was you. This forces the teller to organize his/her recollection of a chain of contacts carefully. It can also help *you* in establishing which of *your* contacts must be notified in case you are infected.

If You Are at the End of a Chain and Are Being Warned

Don't get mad. Appreciate being notified and thank your stars that you have been. And don't alienate your teller; s/he may have some further information at some point that you are going to want to have . . . say, about a "companion" infection. Find out all you can from your teller, but remember that information can get very garbled in stressful circumstances, and you will want to wait for definitive information from your *own* doctor, *after* you have been tested/examined.

Don't get too relaxed about being in the clear just because you are in a place on the chain that makes it unlikely you will also have contracted the infection, or because you have had no symptoms. *And don't dismiss the possibility that* you *may have been the donor, and that you have had a silent case.* **It is always better to be tested/examined than to worry or jeopardize other partners.**

While you are being tested, it can't hurt to be checked out for "companion" infections at the same time. If you find out that you have more than you were informed of, do your teller a favor and let him/her know.

WHAT TO DO IN AN "EXCLUSIVE" RELATIONSHIP

When someone brings a bug into a relationship that is supposed to be sexually exclusive, it's going to mean trouble all around. The thing to keep uppermost in your mind while the two of you are struggling with a disruption that has implications for the core issues of your commitment to each other is the nature and health of that commitment. If revenge or self-righteousness is at the top of your agenda, there will be plenty of opportunity for that; on the other hand, this can also be a chance to make the relationship stronger.

Realize that no matter who is the teller and who the tellee, the information *must* be shared, and that if you are at all committed to each other, you must be committed to getting past this unpleasantness. And before the accusations start flying, you might consider the possibility that one or both of you have been infected but asymptomatic for some time—that is, since before this exclusive relationship began.

Furthermore, teller-tellee lines are blurred in exclusive relationships, both because of guilt and anxiety that are amplified by the intensity of two people who are involved solely with each other, and because if one of you has something and the two of you are regular sex partners the other is likely also to have it . . .

or get it. At any rate, both of you will probably have to be treated as a matter of course, as insurance against ping-ponging, or passing the infection back and forth.

If You Are the One with the Outside Contact

You must tell, of course, because both of you will have to be treated, but tell as gently and lovingly as you can: you must be the one to help your partner adjust to information that is doubly distressing.

Lack of absolute honesty is forgivable, not with the "what" but with the "how." Now is not the time to confess to a string of infidelities, or a heavy involvement with one other person, for that matter. This is adding insult to injury, and your first obligation is to be as supportive of your partner as you can. There are very few of us who cannot conceive of a single and momentary lapse of will that results in a brief encounter, so if it *wasn't* fleeting, it can only help to make it sound as if it was. *This is also not the time for naming names;* emotions are undoubtedly running high. If you haven't been responsible and considerate before, be so now, and think of the other person, who is upset *and* threatened.

If You Are the Offended Party

Don't go crazy. And remember that *sometimes* infections can lurk around for a long time before they reveal themselves. There are also certain infections, like monilia (in women) and prostatitis (in men), that can have suspicious symptoms although they are not necessarily sexually transmitted—meaning that you weren't necessarily "given something." There are other infections, like herpes, that can be latent for a very long time before erupting without any apparent reason. *So be careful what you accuse a loved one of before you have the whole story;* people in sexually exclusive relationships can have a way of jumping to conclusions and being self-righteous, which translates into hysteria and unforgivingness when a sexual infection appears. **If you suspect you have something, *never* fail to tell a significant other because you are afraid of revealing a sexual indiscretion.** S/he has certainly been exposed, and if not treated, will give the infection right back to you. Furthermore, you can seriously threaten his/her health and/or reproductive capacity.

A relationship that breaks up over such an incident is probably less healthy at the moment than you are yourself.

FOR HERPES SUFFERERS

To tell or not to tell? When? How? Whom?

Because genital herpes (HSV-2) has such a stigma attached to it, it is the one sexual infection over which ordinarily responsible and reasonable people go to pieces, either in distress that they may have it—because they feel tainted and untouchable, and fear giving it to someone—or in terror that they might contract it.

There are some things to keep in mind about HSV-2, *aside* from the facts that for the majority of people who get it (and 60% of us have antibodies to it by the age of 21) it will *never* recur after the primary attack, and that for those for whom it does recur more frequently, **herpes should be nothing more than a minor annoyance.** (See the HSV-2 section in Part II for the *rare* exceptions.) These things are:

- There is no *clear* evidence that HSV-2 is communicable when it is *not active.*[1]
- People who *have* HSV-2 *know* when it is becoming active.[2]

This means that:

- Someone who has HSV-2 is both cruel and irresponsible to expose someone who does not.[3]
- Someone who does not have HSV-2 has to be both stupid and irresponsible to be sexually intimate with a partner who has an active lesion.[4]

1. Even in the small number of cases in which it appears that virus is shed *between* perceived periods of activity, it is thought that the concentration of shed virus is too low to communicate the disease.

2. This is called the **prodrome,** a series of symptoms indicating that the virus has been activated, and usually consisting of an itching/tingling/burning sensation in the area—or even on the entire side of the body—in which the lesion will eventually appear. More than 80% of HSV-2 sufferers get very distinct prodromes.

3. There is an exception to this generalization: researchers still are not certain whether a woman who gets vulval *and* cervical lesions can get them at different times (they usually co-occur). Cervical lesions do not announce themselves with a prodrome as consistently as do external lesions of any kind, so a woman *may* have active cervical lesions without knowing it, *if* these lesions have no vulval manifestation.

4. HSV-2 lesions or blisters are quite apparent, especially on the penis. You can see and feel swelling and the sores themselves.

One thing is clear, however, and that is that **an HSV-2 sufferer who has periodic attacks over any number of years can have a complete and satisfying sex life with a partner who does not have HSV-2, and, if s/he is careful, never infect his/her partner.** This means that HSV-2 is not necessarily the heartbreaking disaster it has come to be considered; there are plenty of people in the "frequent outbreak" category who see HSV-2 as nothing worse than a temporary inconvenience about which one must exercise a little good sense. (There has never been much hoopla and hair-tearing about HSV-1—essentially the same syndrome except that it manifests itself orally rather than genitally and means not kissing anyone and not sharing eating utensils, glasses, or lipstick during the few days the sores are active.) **HSV-2 is controllable. HSV-2 does not need to ruin your life.** Having it is distressing enough; you don't have to dismantle your sexual and emotional existence to accommodate it.

If you have HSV-2, therefore, you have a considerable responsibility to be on the lookout for symptoms of the active phase (you may not have recognized the prodrome because you haven't been alerted to it), and *never* take chances on communicating it. (See HSV-2 section in Part II for communicability.) If you have escaped HSV-2 so far, you should never be sexually intimate with a partner who suspects an attack is coming on—even if the blisters have not yet formed—and you should take it upon yourself to check out a partner as well as you can.

Because of its bad reputation, most people who have recurrent HSV-2 are comfortable with *not* telling casual sex partners that they are sufferers—but monitoring themselves carefully. By the same token, HSV-2 sufferers usually *do* tell those with whom they have—or expect to have—an ongoing relationship. As people in general understand more about this disease, the sharing of such personal information will be a less traumatic and painful process than it currently is.

If someone with whom you are involved tells you that s/he has HSV-2, ask him/her whether s/he knows when it is coming on (has a prodrome), where s/he gets it (herpes simplex lesions can be anywhere on the body), and how often. Remember that the person who has told you about his/her HSV-2 feels worse about it than you ever could, and is probably struggling with other complicated responses to it as well. Be thankful your partner has seen fit to be honest with you, and recognize that this indicates that s/he can take and is taking responsibility for having it. HSV-2 sufferers very much appreciate understanding. *And a man can always wear a condom—to protect* either *himself or his partner* —if there is still concern about vulnerability to the virus.

For someone who has caught HSV-2 and is having a primary attack it may help to know that some of the new anti-virals are most effective in just this situation, rather than in recurrences. So if you are unlucky enough to get HSV-2 for the first time—in spite of your caution—get yourself immediately to a doctor so that one of the new therapies can be tried.

SO THIS IS WHY THEY CALL IT A SOCIAL DISEASE

Social diseases come from personal associations, most of them associations that are not limited to sexual encounters. So you want to remember to *let courtesy and consideration rule your behavior in this as it does other areas of your life. When you have to start thinking about the unthinkable, do it calmly.*

In short, be polite. Be kind. Be patient. Don't panic. There's a good chance that sometime in each of our lives, each of us will have to cope with telling . . . or being told.

How to Use This Book... and Notes on Its Contents and Organization

- **This book is meant to educate, not diagnose.** If there is one thing that cannot be said enough, it is that *if you suspect a sexual infection, you must get to a doctor.*

- **Any book built on medical information is only as accurate as the most recent research.** What we know is constantly changing.

- **We have used the term "sexual infection" to denote our subject.** We have chosen this term over "venereal disease" and "sexually transmitted disease" both because "sexual infection" is more inclusive (some of the things we cover are sexually transmitted but not, strictly speaking, venereal, and some are venereal but not necessarily sexually transmitted), and because we think "sexual infection" is a less value-loaded term.

- **We have organized this book according to *category* of infection** (bacterial, viral, etc.), because we think causes and effects are easier to understand when you know something about the organism itself and how it functions. **Within categories, infections are presented in order of frequency of occurrence,** with the most common coming first and the rarest at the end. Please look over the Contents to familiarize yourself with the organization.

- You will find us using some terms that require explanation. **Please read the following section on terms we use** before going further, **and make use of the Glossary** when you need it. There is no reason not to become familiar with proper usage, and you will find our explanations clearer if you know our terminology.

- **There are parts of this book which are repetitive.** This is not a result of poor editing, but rather a response to the likelihood that lots of people will not read this book cover-to-cover, but will look only at sections ... which means that sometimes information is repeated to make sure that even the casual reader is fully informed. (This is especially true in the herpes section.)

- We want to remind you that *every case of every sexual infection is different.* We can tell you the *usual* course of infection, but only a doctor can be sure of what you really have, and then only after clinical confirmation—which usually includes some kind of disagnostic test for the infection-causing organism, without which even a doctor can make a mistake.
- Finally, we haven't written *Healthy Sex* to scare you, but to give you more control over what happens to you sexually.

Terms We Use and Distinctions We Make

The Glossary at the back of this book lists a great many terms in alphabetical order. Here, however, are a few key terms and definitions.

sexual infection   This term is our choice to describe our topic. Not all infections of the sexual parts are sexually transmitted, and not all infections which are primarily of the sexual parts stay there. And "venereal disease" is such an ugly term.

sexually active   Unquestionably you can be sexually active with a single partner, but we have chosen this term to describe someone who has more than a single sexual partner, even if such contacts are rare. "Sexually active" is often used to connote multiple partners. "Promiscuous" should perhaps be left to describe truly extreme activity—joyless, compulsive, indiscriminate sexual coupling.

homosexual men and women   Because the epidemiology of homosexual women does not differ from that of women in general (except that lesbians have a *lower* incidence of all sexual infections than heterosexual women), for the purposes of this book we have made no distinction between gay and straight women.

Gay men, on the other hand, have quite different patterns of sexual—and related—infection from those of straight men (for some diseases); consequently, homosexual men have been addressed in some places as a separate group.

coitus   This is a precise, correct, and convenient word for sexual intercourse—sometimes loosely called just "intercourse." Our language is sadly deficient in useful terms for aspects of sexuality and sexual functioning. (There is no shortage, however, of explicit slang.) Coitus is a good word to know. It is pronounced *ko*-i-tus, with the accent on the first syllable.

ecology   Literally, ecology is the study of environments and the organisms that inhabit them. **Vaginal ecology** is a term you will come across fairly frequently in this book. When we use it we mean the natural balance of microorganisms in the vagina, and what happens when the balance is upset. Some related terms are

flora and **microflora**—literally, the plant life particular to an environment, and here, the organisms that are natural in the healthy vagina—and

organism and **microorganism**—both animal life and plant life, which on the microscopic level in the body include bacteria, viruses, fungi, and protozoa (as well as crabs and scabies, which are not "micro-"). Some microorganisms are

pathogens—These are disease-producing microorganisms, i.e., those microorganisms discussed in this book, among others.

acute/chronic   When said of an infection, **acute** implies intensity and short duration; **chronic** implies long duration and/or recurrence, and a possible resistance to cure.

sore/lesion/ulcer   All are kinds of localized destruction on the surface of the skin or mucous membrane caused by infection by a pathogen. (See Glossary for **lesion** and **ulcer**.)

clinical   An event or thing that can be observed medically is said to be clinical, i.e., when symptoms are present, as in "clinical expression," "clinical picture," and "clinical significance." Therefore, **subclinical** means something that does *not* express itself and is *not* observed, but may be present nonetheless. Subclinical infections by definition do not have symptoms. They can sometimes be detected, however, by the presence of **antibodies** (see below).

immunity   Immunity is the capacity of the body to fight off infection. Those people who do not have this capacity are called **immune-compromised** or **immune-deficient.** Immune deficiencies are either congenital (present at birth) or acquired (because of suppression of natural immunity by drugs or illness).

antibodies   These are special proteins (called **gamma globulins**) manufactured by the body in response to the presence of a foreign substance (called an **antigen**). Antibodies are specific to antigens, and the human body is capable of making thousands of them. Antibodies come from *exposure* to an antigen—or pathogen—so it is possible, if the antigen is a bacterium or virus, for one to have antibodies to a given infection without actually having had clinical manifestations of that infection. This is why with some infections—the herpesviruses, for instance—a much larger proportion of the population has antibodies than has (apparently) had the disease.

Some antibodies confer immunity to the pathogen that caused them. Antibodies in general are the most essential cog in the machinery of the immune system.

Things to Keep in Mind as You Read

- **Sexual infections can happen to anybody. And they do.** Catching a sexual infection does not mean that you are morally corrupt, promiscuous, or unclean—although it is true that the more partners you have, the more likely you are to be exposed to something. Some infections are as common as a cold.
- **Almost everything can be treated, the sooner the better. And by a doctor.** *Do not self-diagnose and self-treat.* Only a doctor knows what you've really got, what to do about it, and when you've gotten rid of it. If you are a woman, *don't* douche before seeing a doctor; it washes away the evidence and makes diagnosis difficult.
- **Sexual infections almost never go away by themselves.** In fact, a symptom that disappears usually suggests just the opposite: that your infection is digging in (where it can make you very sick and interfere with your ability to have children) and becoming harder to diagnose. And to treat.
- **Many sexual infections have *no* symptoms at all . . . especially for women, but also for men.** In other words, there may be no glaring indications that you have something. Therefore you must *stay alert to changes in your own body and be suspicious of anything out of the ordinary in your partner. And on your partner.*
- It used to be that we thought of "venereal disease" and "sexually transmitted disease" as problems that came with sexual intercourse (coitus) only. **In fact, any contact of mucous membrane to mucous membrane—or even skin to skin in some cases—can transmit sexual infection.** However, those that *are* transmitted are usually only spread through *direct contact, although that contact need not be genital.* Most of these organisms are delicate creatures and do not survive for long away from warm wet places *on people,* so it is highly unlikely that a sexual infection is caught from a doorknob or a toilet seat—except under the most extraordinary circumstances. No matter what you'd like to think.
- It also used to be that the idea of "venereal disease" was

limited to syphilis and gonorrhea. **That fact is that by latest count, there are over twenty conditions** (depending on how and what you count) **that qualify as sexual infections**—that is, that show up primarily on the genitals or are transmitted primarily through sexual contact.

- **Not everything that qualifies as a sexual infection is "transmitted,"** so find out what's going on before you go to pieces. Or blame a partner. *Some problems come from a change in body chemistry, or clothes that are too tight, or from nonsexual (albeit human) contact. Some are recurrences of previous infections that have nothing to do with reexposure.* The important thing is to get the proper diagnosis and treatment as soon as possible. Is it worth it to stew?

- **You can have more than one sexual infection at a time. And many people who have one also have another.** It is not uncommon to have a positive culture for gonorrhea before or after syphilis has been diagnosed. HSV-2 (genital herpes), trichomoniasis, and candidiasis frequently co-occur.

    In other words, make sure you are thoroughly checked out for other infections before you are treated for a first one.

- **Get to a doctor—or a clinic—if you even *suspect* a problem, or if you know you have been exposed to something.** Sexual infections are easier to treat in their early stages. And much easier to diagnose, before they "disappear." Only a doctor can be sure if you have picked something up or not. Only a doctor can tell you what to do about it.

- **Nothing is "nothing."** Which is to say that symptoms have causes, and we are finding out that all those "nothings" (nonspecific urethritis in men is the best example) are actually (sometimes serious) *somethings*. Don't accept a "nothing" diagnosis. And don't accept a "blitz" treatment unless you have been told *why* you are getting a blitz rather than being treated for a specific infection. (See the For Women section in Part III especially.)

- Even if you only *suspect* you have something, **spare your partner: never have sexual contact if you think you may have an infection.** You do not need to have *any* symptoms to pass it on.

- **Do not have sexual contact during treatment,** even if you are using barrier contraception, i.e., a condom. What is frequently assumed to be "drug resistance" is more often sim-

35

ple reinfection. This is known as "the ping-pong effect." It is one of the reasons an infection can be so hard to get rid of.

- After being treated, and before resuming an active sex life, **make sure that any and all partners are informed, tested, and—if necessary—treated for what you have been cured of.** *No symptoms in a partner is not the same as no infection.*

- **Always inspect a new partner as well as you can.** This sounds cold, clinical, and difficult to manage, but it *can* be done subtly during sex play. Know what to look for (another reason to educate yourself)—and *look for it.* Sometimes a sensitive touch is worth ten looks. *If you must inquire about a suspicious bump, rash, blister or discharge, don't be shy: DO IT.* (It's your body and your health you are taking chances with.) It may be hell on passion and spontaneity, but it's better than having hell to pay. Sometimes you will have to make eleventh-hour excuses. Let him/her think you are paranoid. So what. (See the For Women and For Men sections in Part III for details on checking out a partner.)

- **You have an obligation to inform any partner(s) if you have a positive diagnosis for a sexually transmitted disease.** (See the earlier section, Sexual Etiquette, for suggestions on how to handle this.) *Any "sin" involved has nothing to do with having the infection and* everything *to do with passing it on when you know you have it.* The information chain must necessarily include a partner who is above you on the chain as well as below—that is, the person who might have given it to you as well as the one *you* infected—and sometimes it is hard to know which is which. (Remember, many infections are asymptomatic, especially in women. A partner may only find out s/he is infected when *you* tell him/her.)
You have a *moral* obligation to inform any partner(s).

Body Maps

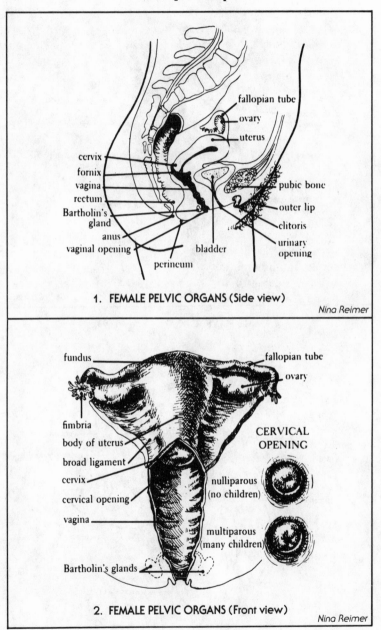

fallopian tube
ovary
uterus

cervix
fornix
vagina
rectum
Bartholin's gland
anus
vaginal opening
perineum
bladder

pubic bone
outer lip
clitoris
urinary opening

1. FEMALE PELVIC ORGANS (Side view)

Nina Reimer

fundus
fallopian tube
ovary

fimbria
body of uterus
broad ligament
cervix
cervical opening
vagina
Bartholin's glands

CERVICAL OPENING

nulliparous (no children)

multiparous (many children)

2. FEMALE PELVIC ORGANS (Front view)

Nina Reimer

37

3. VULVA

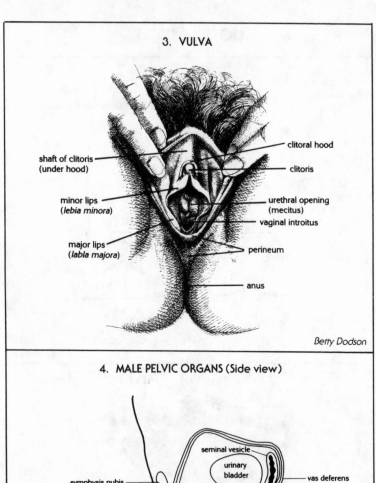

shaft of clitoris
(under hood)

clitoral hood

clitoris

minor lips
(*lebia minora*)

urethral opening
(mecitus)

vaginal introitus

major lips
(*labla majora*)

perineum

anus

Betty Dodson

4. MALE PELVIC ORGANS (Side view)

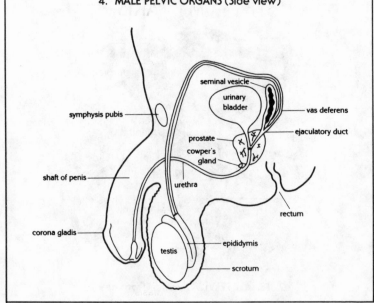

seminal vesicle

urinary
bladder

vas deferens

symphysis pubis

ejaculatory duct

prostate

cowper's
gland

shaft of penis

urethra

rectum

corona gladis

testis

epididymis

scrotum

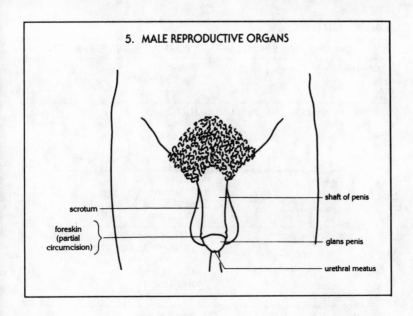

5. MALE REPRODUCTIVE ORGANS

scrotum

foreskin
(partial
circumcision)

shaft of penis

glans penis

urethral meatus

SYMPTOM CHARTS

FOR WOMEN

IF YOU HAVE THIS SYMPTOM	YOU MAY HAVE THIS PROBLEM
vaginal discharge (see discussion of vaginitis in section For Women in Part III)	HV (*Hemophilus vaginalis*) trichomoniasis candidiasis chlamydia gonorrhea HSV-2 (genital herpes)
inflammation and/or itching of the vulva	candidiasis trichomoniasis HV HSV-2 allergic reaction Bartholin's glands infected by gonorrhea
burning during urination	HSV-2 gonorrhea cystitis trichomoniasis candidiasis

FOR WOMEN (cont.)

IF YOU HAVE THIS SYMPTOM	YOU MAY HAVE THIS PROBLEM
swollen labia	HSV-2 infected Bartholin's gland sebaceous cysts
sores or blisters in and/or around the vulva	HSV-2 syphilis occluded hair follicles chancroid granuloma inguinale (rare)
painful coitus	chlamydia trichomoniasis candidiasis endometriosis
lower abdominal pain	PID (pelvic inflammatory disease) from chlamydia or gonorrhea endometriosis ectopic pregnancy ovarian cysts appendicitis

bumps on or around the vulva or perineum	venereal warts
	sebaceous cysts
	occluded hair follicles
	scabies
	syphilis:
	    chancre before it breaks
	    condylomata lata
	molluscum contagiosum
	granuloma inguinale (rarely)

FOR MEN

IF YOU HAVE THIS SYMPTOM	YOU MAY HAVE THIS PROBLEM
discharge from penis	chlamydia (nonspecific urethritis) gonorrhea genital mycoplasmas trichomoniasis E. coli (infection with intestinal bacteria) candidiasis
inflammation of head of penis or urethral opening (meatus), especially under foreskin	candidiasis trichomoniasis gonorrhea
burning during urination	same as **discharge** cystitis

FOR MEN (cont.)

IF YOU HAVE THIS SYMPTOM	YOU MAY HAVE THIS PROBLEM
sores or blisters on and/or around penis	HSV-2 (genital herpes) syphilis LGV (lymphogranuloma venereum) chancroid granuloma inguinale

bumps or growths on and/or around penis	venereal warts
	penile papules
	scabies
	molluscum contagiosum
	syphilis:
	    chancre before it breaks
	    condylomata lata
	granuloma inguinale

lower abdominal pain (including testicles)	chlamydia gonorrhea genital mycoplasmas trichomoniasis

FOR BOTH WOMEN AND MEN

IF YOU HAVE THIS SYMPTOM	YOU MAY HAVE THIS PROBLEM
itching on groin, especially in pubic hair	jock itch (tinea cruris) crabs scabies HSV-2 (followed by pain) candidiasis allergy
anal itch	pinworms or other intestinal infection gonorrhea fungus infection venereal warts
anal pain and/or problems with defecation	HSV-2 (genital herpes) venereal warts intestinal infection hemorrhoids gonorrhea syphilis chlamydia LGV (lymphogranuloma venereum) —in women chancroid
body rash	scabies syphilis (second stage) gonorrhea

IF YOU HAVE THIS SYMPTOM	YOU MAY HAVE THIS PROBLEM
sores on body	scabies HSV-1 or HSV-2 syphilis chancroid granuloma inguinale
sores in or on mouth	HSV-1 or HSV-2 syphilis apthous (see HSV-1) thrush (*candida*)
itchy, gummy eyes	conjunctivitis gonorrhea chlamydia HSV-1 or HSV-2
fever and/or swollen glands	any of the bacterial infections all of the herpesviruses chlamydia, especially LGV genital mycoplasmas

SILENT INFECTIONS AND CARRIERS

Sexual infections that *often have no symptoms* in the **female** but that *can hurt her*—and she can pass on—are:

- **gonorrhea** ⎫
- **chlamydia** ⎬ causes of PID (sterility)
- **syphilis**

Infections that *probably don't hurt her*—and she can pass on—include:

- **genital mycoplasmas**

Sexual infections that *usually have no symptoms* in the **male** that *don't hurt him*—and he can pass on—are:

- **hemophilus vaginalis (HV)**
- **trichomoniasis**

PART II

The Infections

BACTERIAL INFECTIONS

Hemophilus vaginalis • gonorrhea • syphilis • chancroid • granuloma inguinale

BACTERIA
are microscopic, single-cell organisms that are all around us
. . . and in us. Most of the millions of varieties of bacteria are
harmless or even beneficial, but there are some that cause disease, either by producing toxins (poisons) that interfere with the
ongoing life of healthy cells (or even attack them directly and
break them down) or by inciting the body's defenses in the form
of inflammation—pus, redness and swelling, and eventually scar
tissue—which in itself can be very damaging.

A bacterial infection is a process—a process of invasion and
the overwhelming of the body's defenses where the invasion by
the microbe takes place. In this sense, a bacterium is a parasite
of the *body*—a tiny microbe with a definite cell wall and both
nucleic acids, RNA and DNA, unlike a virus. Also unlike a virus, a
bacterium does not need to invade an individual cell to live and
multiply. Antibiotics—which are the agents used against bacterial infections—can attack the bacterium directly, without harming the host, and do their job either by inhibiting bacterial cell
growth or by interfering with its protective outer wall.

The damage done by a bacterial infection may not be apparent
—sometimes there is no inflammation or other visible breakdown of tissues. However, the tissue or body fluid in which it
lives can be sampled and the infection identified, either by microscopic inspection or by growing it in culture.

45

Hemophilus vaginalis (HV)

also coming to be known as *Gardnerella vaginalis,* a commonly occurring vaginal infection caused by *Hemophilus vaginalis* or by *Corynebacterium vaginale*

THINGS YOU NEED TO KNOW

- HV is not serious. It *is* annoying.
- HV is highly infectious.
- Women get HV. Men carry it without knowing it: the organism can be recovered from the urethras of 70–90% of men whose sex partners have HV. Only occasionally will it cause urethritis in the male.
- While HV can be considered to be sexually transmitted, it is also frequently a normal but minor constituent of the flora of the healthy vagina, where overgrowth can be a result of a changing vaginal environment.
- Both partners must be treated to avoid "ping-ponging."
- HV is the organism that has traditionally accounted heavily for a complex of problems that used to be called nonspecific vaginitis. However, as diagnostic techniques are improved this catch-all category (NSV) has become—for treatment purposes—obsolete.

WHERE YOU CATCH IT

Women vagina (vaginitis)
Men urethra (urethritis)

HOW YOU CATCH IT

- coitus with an infected partner, or
- a change in vaginal climate that causes a bacterial imbalance

FIRST SYMPTOMS

appear in about **10 days.**

Women
- a light discharge not related to menstruation that looks and feels like flour paste (gray-white and sticky)
- discharge on the cervix and vaginal walls, and the vagina can have a rashy look
- a red and slightly irritated vulva, which may also itch
- the discharge is likely to have a characteristic strong fishy odor, especially after coitus, because semen reacts with the discharge. This may sometimes be the first indication of infection.

Men
usually have no symptoms, but HV may rarely produce a slight burning or itching on urination, or a slight discharge

WHAT IT DOES

Hemophilus vaginalis colonizes and overgrows in the vagina if the vaginal "climate" is right, so it may be present for a long time before it becomes symptomatic. It is not yet known exactly what the mechanism is, or what circumstances predispose a woman to susceptibility, although it may have to do with a *raised* level of acidity (which is the same as a *lowered* pH). HV causes infection and destruction of surface membranes of the vulva and vagina.

DIAGNOSIS

- HV used to be diagnosed by a process of elimination, but it *does* have a characteristic microscopic appearance, so a doctor should always do a **wet-mount smear.** *Results:* immediate.
- Exposure of vaginal secretions to a drop of potassium hydroxide (10% KOH solution) yields a characteristic fishy smell (called the "whiff test"). This is a simple and generally accurate diagnostic technique, although it is not definitive. *Results:* immediate.
- A culture is done in the case of male infection, and for definitive diagnosis in females. *Results:* 2–3 days.

If you have a vaginal infection, do not douche before seeing your doctor. It washes away the evidence.

TREATMENT

Orally administered <u>antibiotics</u>—especially semisynthetic <u>pen-icillins like ampicillin</u>—are used. Occasionally an agent that is also used for trichomoniasis—Flagyl (metronidazole)—is used.

> <u>It is essential, with any antibiotic, to complete the prescribed course of treatment,</u> even if the symptoms have long since disappeared. Lack of symptoms does not imply a cure, and the cure is not complete until the treatment is. Don't encourage drug resistance with incomplete therapy.

> Women who take antibiotics may develop an annoying vaginal itch. See the discussion of *candidiasis* for prevention and treatment.

THE ALL-CLEAR SIGNAL

- cessation of symptoms, which occurs in about 7 days AND/OR
- completion of prescribed treatment

SPECIAL CONSIDERATIONS FOR WOMEN

Studies indicate that anywhere up to 50% of women (in some samples) who have no symptoms of HV may be colonized by the organism. Usually only the women who develop symptoms need treatment.

Gonorrhea

a surface infection of the mucus-secreting tissues caused by the bacterium *Neisseria gonorrheae*

> BY LAW, THIS INFECTION
> MUST BE REPORTED TO
> THE HEALTH DEPARTMENT.

THINGS YOU NEED TO KNOW

- Gonorrhea is the most common bacterial sexual infection of adults.
- Many—perhaps most—gonorrhea infections have no symptoms . . . until they spread. Of the women who have gonorrhea, probably 90% are unaware of the infection. And as many as 10%—and possibly more—of infected men have no symptoms.
- Lack of symptoms does not mean you cannot infect other people. You can.
- You can also infect yourself in any number of combinations through the discharge: cervix to anus, for instance, or penis to eyes. Or any infected part to any susceptible part.
- The only way to be *sure* you do not have gonorrhea is if you have had a *negative bacterial culture,* and even this is not 100% accurate.
- What is often interpreted as "drug resistance" is simply reinfection from an infected partner who has not been treated concurrently.
- Because gonorrhea has such a short incubation period, it can spread very fast.

WHERE YOU CATCH IT

Gonorrhea is a disease of the mucus-*producing* membranes.

Women   cervix (cervicitis)
                urethra (urethritis)
                Bartholin's glands
Men   urethra (urethritis)
Both
(less commonly)
                anus (proctitis)
                throat
                eyes (conjunctivitis)

HOW YOU CATCH IT

- contact with an infected part
- contact with infected discharge (pus)

GONORRHEA

	LOCAL SYMPTOMS (if any)
MEN urethra	1) discharge of pus from penis 2) burning on urination 3) cloudy urine

WOMEN
    cervix
	1) thick yellowish discharge from vagina
	2) cervical inflammation and/or bumps on cervix
	   (granular erosions)

urethra	1) burning on urination 2) cloudy urine
Bartholin's glands	1) swelling, itching, pain
BOTH anus	1) burning or itching rectum 2) mucus-y stools, or bloody/pus discharge (both rarely)
throat	1) mild sore throat 2) (rarely) severe sore throat
eyes	1) swelling and inflammation 2) pus discharge

FIRST SYMPTOMS

are likely to appear in **3–5 days**—that is, if you *have* symptoms. See the symptom chart.

WHAT IT DOES

The gonococcus organism, transmitted by infected secretions, destroys mucosal cells and stimulates local inflammation and pus (from

COMPLICATIONS	WHAT CAN HAPPEN TO YOU	
	LOCALLY	SYSTEMICALLY
• infection of the prostate and epididymis • testicular involvement marked by swelling, pain and fever • abscesses in urethral glands • infections under foreskin	• damage to sperm ducts • scarring in urethra that can interfere with urination and fertility	
• spread to uterus, fallopian tubes and ovaries, leading to PID (pelvic inflammatory disease) • spread to the peritoneum, the membranous sac covering the abdominal walls and intestines, leading to peritonitis • abscesses involving vital organs, such as liver	• chronic PID, with pain and fever • scarring of fallopian tubes, which can cause sterility and increases the chance of an ectopic (tubal) pregnancy	• infections of the joints (arthritis) • heart and liver infections, which may be fatal • meningitis, which may also be fatal
damage to cornea	blindness	

the white cells that flock to the site). *Local* tissues at the site of infection usually repair themselves with little scarring, but the organism
may persist. Further, the inflamed tissues are vulnerable to secondary
infections by other organisms, like staphylococci or streptococci.
Such secondary infections can permanently impair the function of the
affected organ. In some cases, the gonorrhea becomes systemic, invading the bloodstream and causing serious infections of the joints—
which can result in arthritis—or of the heart, the liver, and the men-
inges—which can kill you.

DIAGNOSIS

- **gram-stain smear,** done in the doctor's office. A drop of pus from a man's infected penis or a woman's cervical secretions is examined under a microscope. This test is of limited usefulness, and is most accurate with urethral gonorrhea in the male. *Results:* immediate, but not diagnostic. Only half of all gram-stain smears can be expected to be accurate enough for diagnosis.

If you have reason to believe that you have been exposed to gonorrhea, and the gram-stain smear is negative, you should have a bacterial culture. Do not have sexual contact until you get the results of the culture.

- **bacterial culture,** taken in the doctor's office and usually sent out to a lab to be grown. *Results:* 2–3 days.

If you have a culture taken, it is best to be cultured *everywhere*—the throat and anus as well as the genitals. A considerable amount of the gonorrhea among teenagers—and homosexuals—is pharyngeal (throat). Gay men also have a high rate of anal infection.

TREATMENT

Gonococcal infections are treated with antibiotics—especially penicillin and its derivatives. If you are allergic to penicillin, other agents can be used. The doctor will decide which drug is best—based on the organism's antibiotic sensitivities and your physical condition, how it is to be administered, and how long it will be used.

> It is essential, with any antibiotic, to complete the prescribed course of treatment, even if the symptoms have long since disappeared. Lack of symptoms does not imply a cure, and the cure is not complete until the treatment is. Don't encourage drug resistance with incomplete therapy.

> Women who take antibiotics may develop an annoying vaginal itch. See the discussion of *candidiasis* for prevention and treatment.

THE ALL-CLEAR SIGNAL

a repeat culture taken 3 to 7 days after completion of treatment. **Do not have sexual contact until you know that this _second_ culture is negative.** If it is positive, consider the possibility that you were reinfected (ping-ponging) or that you have a strain of PPNG (see discussion below).

SPECIAL CONSIDERATIONS FOR WOMEN

- Gonorrhea in women is _usually_ asymptomatic. (A woman who unknowingly passes on a gonococcal infection is known as a _carrier_.)
- **Women who have more than one sexual partner should have themselves cultured regularly—every 3 months or so. Even in exclusive relationships, a culture should be done about once a year.**
- About half the women who have gonorrhea will also have chlamydia.
- About half of all women with untreated gonorrhea will develop pelvic inflammatory disease (PID). (See PID discussion in For Women section, Part III.) There are more than a quarter of a million gonococcal PID cases every year. Even one attack of PID can leave a woman sterile.
- You should have a culture for gonorrhea before having an IUD inserted. And don't forget that an IUD may help gonorrhea ascend from vagina to uterus to fallopian tubes.

SPECIAL CONSIDERATIONS FOR PREGNANT WOMEN

Gonorrhea can blind, damage, or kill a fetus or a newborn who has contracted the infection in the birth canal. A woman should have a culture for gonorrhea as soon as she knows she is pregnant, and continue to have cultures if she has any reason to think she may have been exposed to gonorrhea during pregnancy. By law, all newborns are treated with eye ointments at birth to protect them from gonococcal conjunctivitis, but it is not enough to hope that a partial cure is as good as prevention.

One third of women who have gonorrhea also have group B streptococcus which can be fatal to the newborn. (See discussion of Group B streptococcus in Part III.)

SPECIAL CONSIDERATIONS FOR PARENTS

Children have been known to contract gonorrhea from an infected parent when fresh discharge is on towels, washcloths, hands, or even in the water of a shared bath. For this reason, eye infections or vaginal discharges in infants and small children should be considered suspicious if the child has been exposed to an infected adult.

SPECIAL CONSIDERATIONS FOR MEN

- **First and most important, realize that a woman from whom you've contracted gonorrhea almost certainly doesn't know she has it. You *must* tell any and all female partners that you have the infection, or she/they *may never know.***
- It is not unusual for a man to have a residual discharge after being treated for gonorrhea (post-gonococcal urethritis, or PGU). Originally it was thought that PGU was a reaction to treatment, or some resistant strain of the disease.

    We now know, however, that almost 80% of PGU is really a second infection of chlamydial origin (see the discussion of chlamydia). Chlamydia is frequently contracted at the same time as gonorrhea, and because it is a slower-growing organism that is unresponsive to penicillin, the treatment for gonorrhea does not affect it. For this reason, some doctors now treat gonorrhea with a long course of tetracycline (the treatment of choice for chlamydia) initially.

- About 30% of men who have gonorrhea also have chlamydial infections.

SPECIAL CONSIDERATIONS FOR HOMOSEXUAL MEN

Gay men are epidemiologically at greater risk for gonorrhea because:
- They usually have a higher level of sexual activity—and are active with more partners—than the average heterosexual.
- Anal and throat infections—with less obvious symptoms—are much more common among gays because of the kind of sexual activity they engage in.
- The brief incubation period of the infection makes it more likely that it will be transmitted to one or more partners before the transmitter even knows he has it.

ABOUT PPNG (PENICILLINASE-PRODUCING N. GONORRHEA)

PPNG are strains of gonorrhea—apparently not native to this country—that rather than being eradicated by the usual penicillin treatment for gonorrhea produce an enzyme which breaks down the antibiotic.

PPNG has caused a flap almost on the level of that caused by herpes and by GRID (gay-related immune deficiency, also known as AIDS—acquired immune deficiency syndrome). Here are the facts:
- Contrary to the panic-button press, PPNG *is* curable (spectinomycin is most often used) after being diagnosed with a

special culture—usually after failure of treatment for regular gonorrhea.

- The real threat appears to be small, although it is growing. There were less than 1,000 confirmed cases in 1981—although there were almost 500 in New York City—and that number may double or treble in 1982, with estimates going as high as 1 out of 8 cases of gonorrhea in 1982. There are places where the proportion of PPNG is higher; in the Netherlands, for instance, 20% of all gonorrhea is PPNG.

- PPNG follows clear patterns of spread—from the big cities to the suburbs—that *may* reflect a possible origin: veterans who have served in the Far East and picked up the PPNG there.

- Much of the "resistant" gonorrhea erroneously attributed to PPNG is probably either
  a) chlamydial infection (see discussion of chlamydia), or
  b) reinfection with ordinary gonorrhea from an untreated partner, or
  c) regular gonorrhea incompletely cured because of failure to finish the prescribed course of antibiotics.

Syphilis

an invasive infection progressing from local lesion to systemic disease, caused by the spirochete *Treponema pallidum*

> BY LAW, THIS INFECTION
> MUST BE REPORTED TO
> THE HEALTH DEPARTMENT.

THINGS YOU NEED TO KNOW

- Syphilis can be cured. But left untreated, it can kill you. Or lead to serious progressive disease of the heart, the liver, the nerves and the brain. It can make you crazy. It can paralyze you.

- The infection progresses in three different stages with long intervening periods free of signs or symptoms.
- The First Stage symptom is a primary lesion called a **chancre.** It is painless, and can occur wherever an infected lesion comes into contact with an injured skin or mucosal surface. For all practical purposes—because of minute scratches on these surfaces—this means you can catch syphilis—and get the chancre—anywhere.
- Chancres can be easily mistaken for something else (a pimple, an insect bite, trauma, a herpes lesion) or missed altogether (especially if they are inside the vagina, anus, or mouth). Even doctors can misdiagnose a chancre if inspection is not coupled with testing.
- Second Stage syphilis can have many or few symptoms. These symptoms, as in the First Stage, can look like lots of other things. (Syphilis has been called "the Great Imitator.") 30% of all cases are missed in both Stage One and Stage Two. These cases get picked up in routine screenings—testing for marriage licenses, for example—by accident. It can be a nasty wedding present.
- Syphilis can kill, maim and/or disfigure the unborn child.
- **Masking** of First and Second Stage symptoms can occur if you are being treated with antibiotics for another bacterial infection . . . gonorrhea, for instance. This can be very dangerous. Before you take antibiotics for any other sexual infection, make sure you are screened for syphilis *with a blood test.*
- Diagnosis of Second and Third Stage syphilis can *only* be done by blood test. Treatment requires *prolonged* antibiotic therapy.
- If after you have been cured of a bout with syphilis you are reinfected, you are likely to skip First Stage symptoms altogether, going right into Second Stage.
- If you are sexually active, it is a wise precaution to have a VDRL (blood test) every 6 months.
- Syphilis is one of the few sexual infections that must, by law, be reported to health officials. This is true whether you are treated by a private physician or at a public facility. Their questions are completely confidential, and health officials will contact your sexual partners *for* you—without revealing who you are—if that is more comfortable for you.

- Because syphilis is life-threatening, you must notify any partners (see chart). Consider it wo/manslaughter if you do not notify any and all sexual partners. Because it may be.

WHERE YOU CATCH IT

Syphilis is contracted through the skin where there is an injury —no matter how small. The primary chancre appears at the place in which you came into contact with a lesion. The mucosa is more vulnerable than the skin, but you can get it anywhere.

HOW YOU CATCH IT

by direct contact with the infected part. Organisms do not survive drying or even minor temperature changes.

WHAT IT DOES

An infected lesion transmits the spirochete into damaged skin or mucosa. The organisms quickly spread to the lymph nodes, and 10 to 90 days thereafter a shallow, painless ulcer is formed at the site of inoculation, which is teeming with organisms. The local lymph nodes enlarge but are also usually painless. *The primary chancre goes away by itself.* For variable periods up to 6 months after this there are no signs or symptoms. Until the development of the Second Stage.

Secondary syphilis is characterized most commonly by a blotchy red rash involving any surface—including the palms of the hands and the soles of the feet—loss of hair, and flat lesions—called condylomata lata—on the mucous membrane of the mouth and genitals. (Flat venereal warts—a virus infection—should not be confused with the condylomata lata of syphilis.)

These lesions also go away, after which the syphilis becomes latent, a state which usually lasts for years. During this period the organism does slow but progressive damage to small blood vessels that feed vital organs in all parts of the body. Third Stage syphilis may never occur after this, but if it does, it leads to a weakening and erosion of the aorta (the major artery from the heart), or a degeneration of the brain and the nervous system, resulting in weakness or paralysis, or severe mental disturbances, including psychoses. It can also involve the eyes, the bones, and the liver.

Third Stage manifestations are severely debilitating, often fatal, and incurable. Antibiotics are less effective at this stage, and cannot reverse the damage which has already taken place. A third or more of all people with untreated syphilis will die of some complication of the disease.

SYMPTOMS

- **First Stage** symptom **(chancre)** appears 10 to 90 days after contact. *Average:* **3 weeks.**
- **Second Stage** symptoms appear 6 weeks to 6 months after contact. *Average:* **8 weeks.**

This means that on the average, Second Stage symptoms will appear 5 weeks after First Stage symptoms.

See the symptom chart.

DIAGNOSIS

- **dark-field examination,** done in a doctor's office, or more frequently at a public health clinic, as few physicians have the highly technical equipment for this test. Discharge from the lesion is looked at under a special microscope. Do not clean or medicate the lesion before being tested, or you may compromise its accuracy. Dark-field examination is quite accurate for First Stage syphilis *except* in the case of oral lesions; in fact, early syphilis is much more easily diagnosed by this test, as blood tests at this early stage are accurate only *one third* of the time. In other words, it is worthwhile to find a doctor/clinic that can do this test while your suspicious lesion is still there. *Results:* immediate.

  A blood test may also be done to determine how advanced an infection is, or to diagnose oral lesions.

- **blood test.** The most common blood test—the one you must take by law before you get married—is the **VDRL.** It is one of a class of tests designated *nontreponemal,* which means that it measures antibodies not specific to the syphilis organism. False positive reactions, therefore, are sometimes seen in people with other conditions, like rheumatoid arthritis, or auto-immune diseases. VDRL tests are widely available at health clinics, frequently costing nothing at all, and they are often done first because they are simpler and cheaper than the dark-field test. If you show positive to a nontreponemal test like the VDRL, and there is some question as to whether you actually have syphilis, you will be retested with a *treponemal test* specific to syphilis to be sure of the nature of your infection, and to determine what stage it is in.

Even if the dark-field examination and the blood test are both negative, if you have reason to believe you have been exposed to syphilis, have *another blood test* in a couple of months. More advanced syphilis *always* shows a positive blood test.

It should go without saying that if you have any suspicious sore, or have reason to believe that you have been exposed to syphilis, you *must* refrain from sexual contact of all kinds until you have been seen by a doctor. "Precautions," for all practical purposes, do not exist with syphilis.

TREATMENT

Syphilitic infections are treated with antibiotics—penicillin and certain of its derivatives—in doses which must be maintained for considerable periods of time. *Syphilis is 100% curable in the early stages of the disease.* If you are allergic to penicillin, tetracyclines will probably be used, and if you are pregnant, erythromycin (tetracyclines may discolor the teeth of the fetus). The doctor will determine the schedule on which you receive your medication.

> It is essential, with any antibiotic, to complete the prescribed course of treatment, even if the symptoms have long since disappeared. Lack of symptoms does not imply a cure, and the cure is not complete until the treatment is. Don't encourage drug resistance with incomplete therapy.

> Women who take antibiotics may develop an annoying vaginal itch. See the discussion of *candidiasis* for prevention and treatment.

Anyone treated for syphilis should be aware of the relatively rare phenomenon called the Jarisch-Herxheimer reaction, which can occur within 12 hours of the first treatment. This reaction can make you feel quite ill for a day or so with a new or accentuated skin rash, fever, and headache. Although unpleasant, this

SYPHILIS

		PHYSICAL SIGNS	APPEAR
First Stage	symptoms are recognized only about half the time	• chancre, a firm bump which breaks open into a painless, flat, wet ulcer • swollen lymph nodes, which are usually painless	10–90 days (average 3 weeks) afte contact
Second Stage		• rash, blotchy and red, occurring anywhere on the body, but characteristically on palms of hands and soles of feet	time bet Se
		• mucous membrane involvement: flat lesions in mouth or on genitals; split skin around mouth or nose • patchy hair loss from head, eyebrows, eyelashes • uncommonly: general malaise, with fever, swollen glands, headache	6 weeks to months (average 8 weeks) afte contact Second Sta symptoms may reappe
Latency	no signs or symptoms during this stage (usually uncovered accidentally during routine blood test)		
Third Stage	• weakening of the walls of the aorta (aortic aneurysm)—which may lead to perforation and fatal hemorrhage—or of the heart valves, resulting in heart failure • destructive lesions of the brain or peripheral nerves, leading to meningitis, mental disturbances, psychoses, loss of sensation, weakness, or paralysis • necrotic lesions of organs (e.g., liver) called *gummas* • lesions of the eyes or bones		3–5 years after the primary chancre, or long as 50 years later

LASTS	INFECTIOUSNESS	DIAGNOSIS	EFFECTIVE-NESS OF TREATMENT
3–12 weeks (this means it heals slowly) disappears without treatment	• chancre highly infectious • notify all partners from previous 6 months	• positive diagnosis made by dark-field method • blood tests positive one-third of time	100% if adequate course of antibiotics is prescribed and taken
t and ge: ·ks 2–12 weeks disappears without treatment	• Second Stage skin and mucous membrane lesions are highly infectious • notify all partners from previous year	blood tests always positive	100% with 10–20% retreatment rate
-8 years	syphilis considered to be infectious first 4 years of latency	• blood tests positive • spinal tap	arrests current development, will not reverse damage
r life	not infectious	specialized blood tests are usually positive, but general tests VDRL may be negative	• no effective treatment • no reversal of damage • no changing of course of disease

reaction is dangerous only in advanced cases; the more progressed the disease, the more extreme the reaction.

THE ALL-CLEAR SIGNAL

You should no longer be infectious by about a couple of days following the *completion* of treatment. (Check with your doctor as to when you can resume sexual activity.) However, you should know that it takes quite a while for antibodies to syphilis in your blood to diminish. For this reason—and because it is impossible to know how tenacious any particular case of syphilis may be—**it is important to be retested** on a schedule determined by your doctor to monitor the course of your recovery. **Retesting is the only way to be sure that you are cured.**

SPECIAL CONSIDERATIONS FOR WOMEN

- More than half the women who have syphilis pass through Stage One and Stage Two syphilis without being aware of the disease because
- syphilis chancres are more likely to be hidden in a woman—that is, to be deep in the vagina where she is unaware of them.

SPECIAL CONSIDERATIONS FOR PREGNANT WOMEN

If a pregnant woman has syphilis and is treated before the 4th month of her pregnancy, the infant should suffer no ill effects, because the spirochetes will not have crossed the placental barrier. Even after the 4th month of gestation, there is a good chance that the infant can be cured—*in utero*—when the mother is treated. **However, the rates of spontaneous abortion, prematurity, stillbirth, newborn death, and the deformities of congenital syphilis are very high in *untreated* cases of syphilitic mothers.** For this reason, **every woman should be tested for syphilis (by blood test) as soon as she knows she is pregnant** to pick up silent cases that can cause irreparable harm to the developing baby.

SPECIAL CONSIDERATIONS FOR PARENTS

Congenital syphilis is a particularly horrifying condition. For the babies who survive the first few weeks of life, symptoms are peculiar deformities like saddle nose and holes in the palate, bone lesions and malformations, rash, lesions on the genitals or in the mouth, and nasal discharge. **Almost half of all babies that survive the first few weeks will develop signs of syphilis later.**

- Recently there has been a tremendous rise in the incidence of infectious syphilis among gay men; up to 60% of the cases in urban centers are carried by gays.
- Gay men are much more likely to be unaware of First Stage syphilis because the chancres are frequently in the mouth or the anus.

Chancroid

an acute, invasive infection producing localized destruction of the skin, mucous membranes, and underlying tissue, caused by the bacterium *Hemophilus ducreyi*

> BY LAW, THIS INFECTION
> MUST BE REPORTED TO
> THE HEALTH DEPARTMENT.

THINGS YOU NEED TO KNOW

- Chancroid is hard to miss. It looks awful.
- Chancroid's first symptom (a chancre, which is a painful, spreading ulcer) is much like that of syphilis. The major difference at this stage is that a chancroid lesion is soft, painful, and full of pus. A syphilis chancre is hard, painless, and "clean."
- Chancroid is not as serious as infections that invade the bloodstream, but it can cause considerable local damage.
- Chancroid does not go away unless it is treated. It just gets worse and worse. And uglier and uglier.
- Although chancroid has low infectivity from person to person, it may spread quickly to adjacent tissues on your own self **(auto-inoculation),** especially those places touching the primary ulcer (in skin folds, for instance). It can also spread to—and infect—lymph nodes in the groin.
- Chancroid may co-occur with syphilis, lymphogranuloma venereum (LGV), granuloma inguinale (GI), or herpes (HSV),

and can **mask** any of these. You should be checked for other infections if you have chancroid.

- The organism that causes chancroid is very susceptible to simple soap and water. This means that chancroid can be avoided by good hygiene—especially on moist, covered surfaces that are difficult to clean ... for instance, under a foreskin.
- Chancroid is more likely to occur in tropical climates.

WHERE YOU CATCH IT

the skin and mucosal surfaces of the genital tract; in particular, any protected, moist site.

HOW YOU CATCH IT

- sexual contact with an infected partner
- contact with a lesion

WHERE IT SPREADS TO

- skin of groin area
- lymph nodes in the groin

FIRST SYMPTOMS

are likely to appear in **3–5 days, but may take up to 14 days.** If some damage to the mucosal surface is present at the time of contact, however, a lesion may appear in as little as 24 hours. Asymptomatic cases are relatively uncommon.

WHAT IT DOES

A body surface that has been infected by a chancroid lesion is first colonized and then invaded by *Hemophilus ducreyi*. The result is a deep, painful, purulent ulcer of any size with irregular and undermined edges. The organism may spread to contiguous sites—particularly surfaces touching the original ulcer ("kissing lesions")—and/or to neighboring lymph nodes in the groin, where the painful swelling is a sign of tissue destruction.

Untreated, chancroid utterly destroys affected tissues. Furthermore, drainage from infected lymph nodes may provide an avenue for secondary invasion and systemic infection by other bacteria.

POSSIBLE COMPLICATIONS

- in men: urethritis and a swelling of the foreskin, which can strangle the penis (phimosis)
- for those who engage in anal intercourse: proctitis and anal ulcers
- infected lymph nodes that may need to be drained

DIAGNOSIS

- Chancroid has a very typical **clinical appearance,** so diagnosis is frequently made by sight.
- **bacterial culture** of ulcer taken by a doctor. *Results:* 3–5 days.

TREATMENT

Chancroid is treated with antibiotics—particularly the tetracyclines or erythromycin—or sometimes with cephalosporins. The drugs are administered orally for a week or more.

> It is essential, with any antibiotic, to complete the prescribed course of treatment, even if the symptoms have long since disappeared. Lack of symptoms does not imply a cure, and the cure is not complete until the treatment is. Don't encourage drug resistance with incomplete therapy.

> Women who take antibiotics may develop an annoying vaginal itch. See the discussion of *candidiasis* for prevention and treatment.

THE ALL-CLEAR SIGNAL

complete healing of the ulcer(s)

SPECIAL CONSIDERATIONS FOR WOMEN

Chancroid is frequently hidden in the vagina in women and may progress more slowly. Painful urination (or defecation in the case of an anal infection) are often presenting symptoms.

SPECIAL CONSIDERATIONS FOR MEN

Chancroid is more common in uncircumcised men.

SPECIAL CONSIDERATIONS FOR HOMOSEXUAL MEN

Chancroid can be hidden in the anus. Painful defecation may be a symptom.

Granuloma Inguinale

a relatively rare, locally invasive infection caused by the bacterium *Donovania granulomatatis,* which incites a destructive inflammatory lesion called a granuloma

> BY LAW, THIS INFECTION
> MUST BE REPORTED TO
> THE HEALTH DEPARTMENT.

THINGS YOU NEED TO KNOW

- Granuloma inguinale (GI) is a rare disease occurring almost exclusively in people who live in hot, humid climates (in the United States, this means the Southeast), although there was a recent epidemic in Greenland.
- GI has low communicability—that is, it is not easy to catch.
- GI is a slow-growing infection that takes anywhere from 1 to 12 weeks to develop.

- GI is chronic and <u>causes permanent scarring.</u> This holds true even after it is cured. (The scar is characteristically hard and deeply pigmented.)
- It is not absolutely clear that the mode of transmission is sexual, even though the disease is classified as venereal because the lesion appears on sexual parts.

WHERE YOU CATCH IT

Women   labia of the vagina . . . but it can appear on the buttocks or perineal skin
Men   penis: glans or shaft

HOW YOU CATCH IT

by direct <u>contact</u> with a granuloma lesion

SYMPTOMS

may be **slow to appear** (1–12 weeks). The first sign is a small blister or red lump which slowly enlarges and erodes to form an ulcer with raised edges. In the early stages the lesion is painless but it may *become* painful and secondarily infected.

WHAT IT DOES

The organism invades tissues through the skin following direct contact and incites a slow, chronic, destructive inflammatory response called a granuloma. This inflammatory response is a mix of large white cells which engulf and restrict the growth of the organism. These large inflammatory cells also kill normal tissues, producing ulceration and promoting scarring which limits the spread of the infection. GI rarely occurs on other parts of the body, although it may infect the bones, resulting in a chronic destructive bone condition called osteomyelitis.

DIAGNOSIS

by microscopic examination of infected tissue (tissue smear) for a characteristic bacteria formation called a Donovan body

TREATMENT

GI is treatable, but requires <u>long antibiotic therapy</u> and resolves slowly.

THE ALL-CLEAR SIGNAL

When the lesion has healed and scarred over, and the inflammation has disappeared, the infection is gone.

INTERMEDIATE ORGANISMS

chlamydia • genital mycoplasmas

INTERMEDIATE ORGANISMS
are so called because they have characteristics both of bacteria and of viruses. They are smaller than bacteria, and, like bacteria, they are "complete" organisms because they have both RNA and DNA. They can live outside of the human cell.

To multiply, however, they must—like viruses—invade and take over a cell. And like viruses, they have no defined structural wall.

Intermediate organisms are susceptible to antibiotics, which inhibit their growth.

Chlamydia

actually a series of related infections caused by the
"intermediate" organism *Chlamydia trachomatis*

THINGS YOU NEED TO KNOW

- Chlamydia is epidemic in the United States: it may occur as much as three times as frequently as gonorrhea in men, and between five and ten times as often as gonorrhea in women.
- Chlamydial infections are highly contagious.
- You may not have heard of chlamydia yet, but although the name is new, the complex of infections the organism causes is old. Probably more than half of what used to be called nonspecific urethritis (NSU)—or nongonococcal urethritis (NGU)—in men is caused by *C. trachomatis*. (There are currently as many as *2.5 million* cases of NGU.) Furthermore, as many as 30% of men with gonorrhea also have chlamydia, which may show up as what used to be called *postgonococcal urethritis (PGU).* By the same token, much difficult-to-diagnose-and-cure vaginitis—as well as a high proportion of PID—is the result of chlamydial infections. As many as half the women with gonorrhea will also have chlamydia, which may show up as postgonococcal cervicitis.
- Chlamydial infections tend to develop slowly and to be associated with relatively mild symptoms. But just because they develop in subtle ways does not mean that they cannot cause significant destruction to involved tissues.
- In countries that keep figures on chlamydial infections (which the United States is just beginning to do, usually under the category of nongonococcal urethritis in men), the organism has been blamed for anywhere from 50% to 90% of the pelvic inflammatory disease (PID) in women. (See PID in the For Women section in Part III.) Chlamydial PID is also more likely to result in scarring of the fallopian tubes—which can result in infertility and tubal (ectopic) pregnancy —than gonorrhea-caused PID.
- Chlamydial infections have serious implications for the pregnant woman and the newborn child. A baby born to an

infected mother is at high risk for developing an eye infection (conjunctivitis) that can result in blindness (worldwide, *trachoma* is the most common cause of blindness), or a pneumonia that can result in death.

- Chlamydial infections are associated with a number of serious complications if left untreated, including

>*sterility:* from PID in women
>
>>from epididymitis in men
>
>*Reiter's syndrome:* a debilitating co-occurrence of urethritis, arthritis, and conjunctivitis
>
>*lymphogranuloma venereum:* a rare venereal disease (there is a discussion of LGV later in this section)

WHERE YOU CATCH IT

Women cervix (cervicitis), spreading to
fallopian tubes (salpingitis) and
urethra (urethritis)
potentially the peritoneum (peritonitis)

Men urethra, spreading to the epididymis (epididymitis)

Infants eyes (conjunctivitis)
upper respiratory tract
lungs (pneumonia)

HOW YOU CATCH IT

Adults are infected through sexual intercourse. Infants are infected during vaginal delivery.

SYMPTOMS

are **slow to appear,** with a large number of asymptomatic cases. Technically, the incubation period is **3 weeks.**

Women
- occasionally a slight discharge
- pain during coitus (dyspareunia)
- chlamydial infections are frequently diagnosed in their later stages, when they present as slowly developing lower abdominal pain and fever, although the symptoms are likely to be less severe and clear-cut than with gonorrhea

Men
- pain on urination
- urethral discharge

WHAT IT DOES

Chlamydia trachomatis invades and replicates in mucus-producing and other secretory cells lining the genital tract. It then spreads to deeper tissues, where it stimulates a slowly developing but destructive inflammatory response that can finally manifest itself almost anywhere in the body.

In **women,** the infection is frequently asymptomatic, although it is likely to pass from the vaginal tract and cervix to the lining of the uterus (endometritis) and from there to the fallopian tubes (salpingitis). It may further pass to the peritoneal cavity (peritonitis, and pelvic inflammatory disease or PID). The infection may eventually progress to the surface of the liver.

In **men,** the infection may extend from the urethra to the epididymis (epididymitis), where it can result in sterility.

In **both sexes,** certain strains of *C. trachomatis* can invade the lymph nodes—producing a condition highly destructive to these glands and their surrounding tissue called *lymphogranuloma venereum*—and from there spread to the rest of the body, particularly in people who may have lowered resistance. In such people other severe infections, like pneumonia, may develop.

The organism has a high likelihood of being cultured from the partner of someone who is already infected. This means that **if your partner has it, you are likely to have it too (or vice versa) even though there are no symptoms.**

SOME CONDITIONS ASSOCIATED WITH *C. TRACHOMATIS*

trachoma
paratrachoma
urethral syndrome
Fitz-Hugh Curtis syndrome
bartholinitis
postpartum endometritis
proctitis
Reiter's syndrome
lymphogranuloma venereum
salpingitis
epididymitis
perihepatitis

adult pneumonia
pelvic inflammatory disease
endocarditis
spontaneous abortion
infant conjunctivitis
infant pneumonia
sudden infant death syndrome
otitis media
prepubertal vaginitis
cervicitis
pharyngeal infections
peritonitis

DIAGNOSIS

- **by specialized culture,** not usually available in a doctor's office, or to the labs that serve private physicians. The specialized cultures which give a definitive diagnosis are most likely to be available in well-equipped VD clinics, or in hospitals. Routine culturing is currently prohibitively expensive, but new techniques are being developed. If we are lucky, they should be available soon.
- In the absence of a convenient and easy diagnostic tool, *diagnosis is often made by the process of elimination: if* all the clinical signs of a chlamydial infection are present, and a culture demonstrates no other infection, chlamydia is deduced. Deduction is also used in the case of men, when gonorrhea has been ruled out in cases of urethritis. (Almost all nongonococcal urethritis is chlamydial in origin.)

It is often safer to assume *chlamydia and treat for it than be sorry.*

TREATMENT

Even though chlamydial infections are not caused by bacteria, the current treatment of choice is antibiotics: tetracyclines and sulfonamides, taken orally. Because of their extended incubation periods, *these infections must be treated for up to 3 weeks.* (This is the reason that penicillin treatment for gonorrhea is not adequate to eradicate the slower-developing *C. trachomatis.* It is also why more gonorrhea is now being treated initially with tetracyclines.) It may also be that a large proportion of the "penicillin-resistant" gonorrhea (PPNG), as well as PGU, or postgonococcal urethritis, is really chlamydia that has been contracted at the same time as the gonorrhea.

Treating partners is *essential* to avoid ping-ponging.

It is essential, with any antibiotic, to complete the prescribed course of treatment, even if the symptoms have long since disappeared. Lack of symptoms does not imply a cure, and the cure is not complete until the treatment is. Don't encourage drug resistance with incomplete therapy.

Women who take antibiotics may develop an annoying vaginal itch. See the discussion of *candidiasis* for prevention and treatment.

THE ALL-CLEAR SIGNAL

- cessation of symptoms
  and/or
- completion of drug therapy

ABOUT LYMPHOGRANULOMA VENEREUM

SPECIAL CONSIDERATIONS FOR WOMEN

- Chlamydial infections are particularly insidious in women because their symptoms are subtle *(perhaps 75% of cases are asymptomatic),* and the **infections can progress to full-blown pelvic inflammatory disease (PID) with very little indication of that progression.** For this reason, lower abdominal pain and fever should always be considered a possible sign of chlamydia-induced PID. (Don't forget that gonorrhea also causes PID.)
- Chlamydia-induced PID is more likely to cause scarring . . . and consequently more likely to interfere with fertility, as well as to put a woman at higher risk for a tubal (ectopic) pregnancy. Research indicates that probably half of all ectopic pregnancies occur in women who have a history of PID.
- **C. trachomatis is the most frequently isolated sexually transmitted organism found in women who attend clinics that are prepared to test for it.** This means that a woman with an infection is more likely to have chlamydia than anything else. In one study (in Sweden, where they routinely test for chlamydial organisms) 80% of women with blocked tubes had chlamydial antibodies, and *50% had current infection.*
- *C. trachomatis* is associated with "cervical pathology." Whether the organism is responsible for such pathology—or simply more welcome where such pathology already exists—is not clear.

SPECIAL CONSIDERATIONS FOR PREGNANT WOMEN

- It is hard to overemphasize the damage that chlamydia can do to the newborn.
- *C. trachomatis* has been implicated in premature delivery.
- Women who have chlamydia are twice as likely as other women to develop childbirth (puerperal) fever. Almost one third of mothers with chlamydial infections during pregnancy will develop it.

SPECIAL CONSIDERATIONS FOR MEN

Men should be aware that it is one of the chlamydial organisms that is responsible for lymphogranuloma venereum (LGV), a highly destructive infection of the lymph nodes and surrounding tissues. Men are at higher risk for this infection than women. Invasion is by way of urethral infection.

SPECIAL CONSIDERATIONS FOR HOMOSEXUAL MEN

Aside from the risk of LGV, homosexual men may have another manifestation of *C. trachomatis:* anal infections (proctitis), in which scarring in the bowel wall may lead to obstructions.

> BY LAW, THIS INFECTION
> MUST BE REPORTED TO
> THE HEALTH DEPARTMENT.

LGV is a highly contagious infection of the lymph nodes caused by one strain of *C. trachomatis.* Men are more likely to catch it . . . *and* have clear symptoms of it. It starts with a little pimple or sore on the genitals that may not be noticed and then goes away by itself, usually within a week. The next symptom—in men—is usually swollen glands in the groin; in women it is usually internal swelling around the rectum that can cause rectal strictures and is often blamed on something else. It progresses to flu-like symptoms, with chills, fever, and body aches, and in its later stages is highly destructive of the lymph nodes and surrounding tissue.

LGV is diagnosed with specialized blood tests, and treated with sulfonamides. The infection resolves slowly, taking 3 weeks to a month to disappear completely.

It is unclear just how long the incubation period is, but it is probably about a week.

Genital Mycoplasmas

intermediate organisms (previously called pleuropneumonialike organisms, or PPLO, and sometimes called ureaplasmas) that are a frequent normal inhabitant of the genitourinary tract, and include *Mycoplasma hominis* (also known as *Ureaplasma hominis*) and *Urea urealyticum* (also known as *T. mycoplasma*)

THINGS YOU NEED TO KNOW

- Information about genital mycoplasmas and their effects on people is very incomplete. It is thought, however, that it is probably only *U. urealyticum* that causes a sexual infection, and then usually only in men.
- The presence of the organisms and their concentration seem to be in proportion to sexual activity. This means that the more sexual partners you have, the more likely you are to have mycoplasmas in your genital tract.
- *U. urealyticum* can cause urethritis and sometimes prostatitis in men; women—while they often harbor the organisms —appear to be unaffected by them, except in rare cases.

WHERE YOU CATCH THEM

the mucous membranes of the entire genitourinary tract

HOW YOU CATCH THEM

coitus

SYMPTOMS

M. hominis appears to have no symptoms. Those of *U. urealyticum* are apparent in men.

Women rarely symptomatic; mycoplasma is usually an incidental finding when other pathogens are present

Men
- urethritis (inflammation and discharge)
- prostatitis
- flu-like fever and aches

WHAT THEY DO

The course of an infection with mycoplasma is as yet unclear; neither do researchers know what effects an infection may have.

DIAGNOSIS

by specialized culture, not likely to be available in a private physician's office. These are fragile organisms and grow only under well-controlled circumstances.

TREATMENT

Genital mycoplasmas are treated with <u>tetracyclines</u> when they *are* treated; however, since so little is known about them, antibiotics are given only when they actually cause an infection. In this case the (usually female) sexual partner must also be treated to avoid reinfection.

THE ALL-CLEAR SIGNAL

- when the course of treatment is completed (for both partners)

AND/OR

- when the symptoms have gone away

STAY POSTED

Mycoplasmas are getting much research attention right now (you can probably tell that just by how many names they have), and we are likely to know a great deal more about them in the future.

SPECIAL CONSIDERATIONS FOR PREGNANT WOMEN

Mycoplasmas have been implicated in infertility, spontaneous abortion, prematurity, and stillbirth, but there is no real proof of this apparent connection.

SPECIAL CONSIDERATIONS FOR MEN

Your female partner hasn't "burned" you if you are diagnosed as having mycoplasma: it is often a usual inhabitant of the vaginal tract to which some men are sensitive. But if you *are* sensitive, you must be sure that your partner is treated when you are, or your urethritis will come back.

VIRAL INFECTIONS

*herpesvirus: herpes simplex type 1, herpes simplex type 2,
cytomegalovirus, Epstein-Barr virus • venereal warts • molluscum
contagiosum • (viral hepatitis is discussed under FOR GAY MEN)*

VIRUSES

are submicroscopic organisms (indeed, they are so small that
they can be seen only with an electron microscope and are
sometimes regarded as complex proteins rather than organisms)
that can cause disease in living things. They have a *single* nucleic acid—either RNA or DNA (unlike bacteria, which have both)
—and neither a cell wall nor any internal cellular machinery for
metabolism or reproduction.

"Free" viruses, therefore, are a threat only when they invade a
living cell; they are parasites that live and multiply by borrowing
the cell's machinery and commandeering it—a sort of body-
snatcher—usually causing, in the process, the degeneration and
finally the destruction of that cell.

While medicine has developed a large battery of antibiotics to
control bacterial infections, it has not done so well with viral
infections. Most antiviral agents work by interfering with viral
replication (via its genetic material); however, these drugs often
interfere with the replication of normal cells as well, resulting in
toxicities which limit their use to life-threatening infections
where the risk of toxicity is outweighed by the seriousness of the
viral infection. The recent development of drugs which are effective in life-threatening herpesvirus infections has provided drug
models that have possibilities but need to be improved upon;
nevertheless, it shouldn't be long before we have safe agents for
the control of minor local viral infections.

Herpesviruses—In General

Everyone "knows" about herpes, but very few of us know enough. No other class of sexually transmitted diseases has caused so much confusion, spawned so much misinformation, and been at the root of so much needless anguish as this family of infection-causing organisms.

Herpesviruses and their manifestations are to be found in every kind of animal, not just human beings. Human beings are susceptible to five different herpesviruses, four of which can be sexually transmitted, with two of these—the herpes simplex viruses Type I and Type II—being closely related.

There are some basic facts that apply to *all* human herpesvirus infections:

- **There is as yet no effective cure for any herpesvirus infection,** although some new antivirals are successful in limiting or reversing symptoms of the active phase of the diseases caused by these viruses.
- **All herpesviruses share a latency characteristic:** once you have contracted them, you have them, although the virus may not be active. At least three herpesviruses are known to be able to recur spontaneously: the two herpes simplex viruses, and varicella-zoster (chicken pox, which recurs as shingles in adults).
- **The great majority of people have antibodies to all five herpesviruses** (see chart). "Having antibodies" is evidence of prior exposure and infection, whether the symptoms were apparent or not.
- **The five human herpesviruses do not constitute a significant health risk except in rare cases.** The two consistent—and considerable—medical concerns are the apparent rela-

tionship between herpesviruses and some kinds of cancer, and the threat active infections pose to the fetus and newborn.

The four herpesviruses which can be sexually transmitted are:

- **herpes simplex virus Type I (HSV-1),** also known as *herpes labialis* because it is commonly associated with "cold sores" or "fever blisters" on the mouth and lip
- **herpes simplex virus Type II (HSV-2),** also known as *herpes progenitalis* because of its common association with genital lesions
- **cytomegalovirus,** best known for its threat to the fetus—as a cause of birth defects and infant mortality—and for its possible relationship to a malignancy being seen more frequently among homosexual men
- **Epstein-Barr virus,** the proper name for the virus that causes infectious mononucleosis

The fifth herpesvirus—which is *not* sexually transmitted—is:

- **varicella-zoster,** or chicken pox, to you. This is the same herpesvirus responsible for shingles in later life.

THE TWO HERPES SIMPLEX VIRUSES: HSV-1 AND HSV-2

DNA-containing viruses of the herpesvirus family, distinguished from each other by specific antibodies and their DNA "maps"

Type I or **herpes labialis** is associated with lesions on the mouth and lips ("cold sores" and "fever blisters"). It is a very common infection that most people are exposed to—and contract—before puberty. It is usually transmitted orally rather than genitally, and so is not—in the strictest sense—a venereal infection.

Type II or **herpes progenitalis,** distinguished relatively recently from HSV-1, is identified with genital lesions and venereal transmission.

However, while it is true that the *majority* of HSV-1 infections are found above the waist, and the *majority* of HSV-2 infections are found below it, there is considerable crossover owing to changes in sexual practices: HSV-1 can infect the genitalia (as well as the nipple and other skin surfaces), and HSV-2 has been cultured with increasing frequency from lesions on—and, if it's a primary attack, in—the mouth. Many medical observers feel that this growing rate of crossover will soon obliterate the original structural distinctions between HSV-1 and HSV-2, and that herpes simplex infections will come to be identified primarily by the site of the lesion: oral or genital.

For reasons of clarity and brevity for this book, we have adopted the convention of referring to *HSV* when we mean *both* infections and are discussing aspects of them that are functionally alike, to *HSV-1* when we mean the herpes simplex virus associated with the common "cold sore"; and to *HSV-2* when we mean the lesions that appear on and around the genitals (including the buttocks and thighs). As per the above explanation, this does *not* imply that either infection is restricted to specific parts of the body.

However, this *also* does not mean that if you have an attack of *genital* herpes your *saliva* is infectious . . . or that if you have a cold sore you may not have coitus (although you wouldn't have oral-genital contact). A herpes virus *attack* means <u>you are infectious only at the blister site.</u>

THE "TERRIBLE CURSE" OF HERPES

In the last year, the flood of attention to herpes (and when "herpes" is mentioned, people almost always are referring exclusively—and inexactly—to genital herpes) has all but swept away every vestige of good sense, scaring the wits out of both the people who don't have it and the people who do. Headlines about "heartbreak" and "curses" and "the new scarlet letter" put herpes infections—and, by association, all sexual infections—in a spotlight that does little to illuminate this health problem. People can't be expected to behave sensibly and responsibly, or to react calmly, when they are bludgeoned with innuendo and outright misinformation.

Here are two important *facts* about herpes:

- **Herpes does not constitute a significant health risk to normal adults, except in very rare cases (unlike some other sexual infections, which *can* kill you).**

- **While herpes is incurable, so are—in the *same* sense— cold sores and chicken pox.** And we don't spend much time obsessing about our incurable HSV-1 and varicella zoster . . . although both are as likely—or *more* likely—to recur than HSV-2.

The mundane fact is that with perhaps *twenty million* cases of genital herpes (that is one out of five American adults) and another half million being added annually, the horror stories belong to the very few rather than the many. Most people with genital herpes have learned to live with it as people of earlier generations have accommodated the occasional cold sore (caused by HSV-1) or attack of shingles (varicella zoster). It is instructive to consider, for instance, how long Western civilization has managed to live with the latter two nuisances without the uproar and moral indignation that surrounds the man/woman

HERPESVIRUS STATISTICS

HERPES-VIRUS		% OF POPULATION WITH ANTIBODIES INDICATING PRIOR INFECTION	% OF INFECTED POPULATION WITH **SINGLE** OCCURRENCE OR VERY RARE RECURRENCE	% OF INFECTED POPULATION WITH **MULTIPLE** RECURRENCES
HSV-1	lesion	95% by age 17	30–50%	5–10%
HSV-2	lesion	60–80% by age 21	approximately 60%	5–10%
CMV		60–80% by age 40; 90% among male homosexuals	Unknown: while active infection may recur, it is frequently asymptomatic and usually resolves spontaneously.	
E-BV		85% by age 15		
V-Z	lesion	virtually 100% (chicken pox)	80% (shingles)	3–5%

(may be sexually transmitted)

with genital herpes—with its attendant feelings of punishment, guilt, self-loathing, and depression.

In view of this, one can't help postulating that we are less concerned about genital herpes per se than about its mode of transmission and the geography of its manifestations—both sources of considerable and long-standing anxiety to most "nice" people—who may be having the first and only run-in they will ever have with a sexual infection when they contract HSV-2.

One of the ironies of HSV is that perhaps the most consistent activating factor of the virus in most of the people who suffer recurrent attacks is *emotional stress.* This fact fits neatly with the developing epidemiology of HSV-2, which is exploding in the well-educated middle-class segment of the population—the same "clean," cautious, frequently puritanical middle class that reflexively makes subtle connections between moral laxity and appropriate punishment.

It follows, then, that the first thing to do is **stay calm.** Unless you are an immune-compromised person or a newborn, HSV is not going to kill you, and getting crazy is exactly the thing likely to make you more vulnerable to recurrences. Millions of people infected with HSV have active, healthy sex lives, and *never* transmit the disease to a sex partner.

THINGS YOU NEED TO KNOW ABOUT BOTH HSV-1 AND HSV-2

- HSV-1 does not confer immunity to HSV-2, and vice versa. Neither does a particular strain (and there are a number of strains) confer immunity to other strains, although it is *unlikely* that you would catch another strain.
- **Once you have been infected** with HSV-1 or HSV-2, **the virus can persist in the body indefinitely.**
- **Only a small fraction of previously infected people will have recurrences**—that is, only relatively rarely will the virus be reactivated and produce symptoms.
- **Recurrence of symptoms** in previously infected people **almost never reflects a new exposure, but rather reactivation of old infection.**
- **HSV recurrences** (both 1 and 2) are poorly understood, but **are thought to be triggered by either physical trauma or**

emotional stress. Physical trauma includes sunburn (and ultraviolet light), local irritation, fever or other infections, and the use of drugs which compromise resistance. How emotional stress encourages recurrences is not yet clear; however, it may be related either to central nervous system excitation (centrally controlled), or to some chemical modulation of the immune system associated with mood change. (Did you ever notice how much more likely you are to get sick with *anything* when you are under stress?)

- **HSV attacks are** almost always **self-limited. Primary infections** (both oral and genital) **are likely to be more severe—** and last longer—**than subsequent attacks** . . . if there are any. (See the herpesvirus chart.)

- **There is** presently **no cure for HSV,** although there are effective antivirals which can be administered systemically for life-threatening infections. These antivirals, when used topically, *may* give *some* symptomatic relief and speed resolution of local infection.

- HSV lives in the sensory nerve cells of the brain or spinal cord, where it remains indefinitely, causing problems only when it is activated. Physical, emotional, and—probably— hereditary factors determine susceptibility to activation, and the **frequency of recurrence is no reflection of either sexual practices or the number of sexual partners.**

- Many people who have HSV-1 and HSV-2 know when an attack is imminent because of the **prodrome**—burning, itching, tingling, or aching sensations in the area where the lesions from the activated virus will appear.

- As a working rule, **HSV is likely to be contagious only when —and where—it is active.** For example, although periodic shedding of HSV-1 virus can be detected in the saliva of about 10% of those previously infected (even if there are no detectable lesions), it is not established that either the concentration or the character of this shed virus is such as to be infectious to someone else.

- **Active lesions of HSV are,** on the contrary, **highly infectious. Virus is shed from a lesion for an average of five days,** with the greatest amount shed on the second day of an attack.

COMPLICATIONS SHARED BY HSV-1
AND HSV-2

- **HSV infection of the eye**—herpes keratitis or ocular herpes—is usually a complication of oral herpes, but active virus can be carried to the eye—where it attacks the tissues overlying the cornea—from anywhere. Herpes keratitis is the leading cause of *infectious* blindness in the United States. Fortunately, this is one type of HSV which is responsive to antiviral drugs if it is recognized early enough. If you have active HSV *anywhere,* keep your hands clean and away from your eyes, and *never* use saliva to wet contact lenses.

- **Immunologically compromised people—including newborns, those receiving cancer chemotherapy, people who are malnourished, and those suffering from immune-deficiency diseases (as well as *rare* otherwise normal individuals)—are vulnerable to severe HSV infections, which may become systemic . . . and lethal.** Systemic manifestations include encephalitis, meningitis, esophagitis and tracheal infections, pneumonia, and hepatitis.

- Extensive **spread of local infection may** also **occur** where skin is already damaged **with eczema.**

- There is always the possibility of **secondary bacterial infection** where a lesion or blister has been scratched or picked. In the case of the immunologically compromised, such secondary infection may become blood-borne.

WHERE YOU CATCH HSV

just about anywhere, with the majority of Type I infections being above the waist, and a majority of Type II below it. Mucous membranes are very susceptible to invasion, but any skin surface is a potential site for a lesion. That is, any place on the body can transmit HSV to any other place.

HOW YOU CATCH HSV

contact with an active lesion, or with the fluid from the lesion, which is swarming with active virus. Virus can be transported from one site to another by the hands. The eye is especially vulnerable.

SYMPTOMS

appear anywhere from 2 to 20 days after exposure, although they can develop within 24 hours. The **average is 6 days.**

Recurrent HSV infections are often heralded by the **prodrome** —tingling, itching, burning, or aching sensations in the general area of the prior outbreaks. The prodrome lasts from 6 hours to 2 days, when swelling begins, with small blisters—usually grouped together—forming on the swelling. At this point discomfort often localizes to the site of the infection, and the prodrome may dissipate.

The blisters break open and drain in the course of the attack, leaving open ulcers which scab over and heal completely.

It is unusual for secondary attacks to be in different places than the primaries, although they may relocate slightly in the neighborhood of the infected nerve cells. If a lesion appears in a totally unexpected place, however, consider the possibility that it is not caused by HSV. (Alternatively, it *may* be caused by reinfection with another strain.)

WHAT IT DOES

The herpes simplex virus infects the surface cells at the initial point of contact, killing them, and in the process producing many progeny. The new virus derived from the surface lesion will then invade sensory nerve cells serving the primary site of infection, passing up the nerve fiber to the nucleus of the cell in the spinal column or brain. HSV does *not* kill the nerve cell but remains dormant in it. Undue stimulation of the sensory nerve—either physical stimulation at the original site, or central nervous system stimulation in the form of psychological stress —may reactivate the virus (or possibly alter the carrier's resistance), so that the virus again passes down the nerve fiber and reinfects the overlying surfaces (skin or mucosa), producing a secondary lesion.

DIAGNOSIS

- by **inspection.** Clusters of small painful or itchy blisters are typical for HSV lesions (see the later discussions of HSV-1 and HSV-2 for specifics). However, there are other conditions/diseases that are characterized by blister-like eruptions (canker sores, syphilitic chancres, and certain autoimmune disorders are only a few examples) on mucosal surfaces in the mouth *and* on the genitals, and HSV infections are all too frequently misdiagnosed.

- A suspicious lesion can only be *absolutely identified* by **culture,** grown from a sample scraped from the base of an open blister. In addition, such cells may be markedly enlarged, with multiple nuclei—a characteristic of HSV which can be seen with a microscope.
- Presumed diagnosis can be made if HSV-2-specific antibodies develop when none existed before.

TREATMENT

HSV infections and their recurrences are generally self-limited and resolve over a period of 3–10 days. Certain new antiviral agents (see below) may shorten the period of pain and blistering and are clearly effective in treating infections which occur in the eye. (These preparations have little impact on oral and genital HSV.)

It should be stressed that administration of topical antiviral agents—while *possibly* shortening the duration of local infections and relieving pain—do not eradicate the virus from nerve cells and therefore do not "cure" the infection. Recurrences after treatment almost always represent reactivation of the virus latent in the nerve cell.

THE NEW ANTIVIRAL DRUGS

- **Acycloguarosine** (ACG or Acyclovir) has been found—*in certain studies*—to be useful in the treatment of skin lesions, shortening the symptomatic period as well as the period of viral shedding (thereby reducing the possibility of infecting someone else). Used against skin lesions, it is most effective in a primary attack and is probably ineffective in subsequent ones.

  ACG does not kill the virus, but does prevent the number of "commandeered" cells from increasing. Like most antivirals, ACG is a relative of anti-cancer drugs which can be extremely toxic to dividing cells such as blood cells.

  ACG has not yet been licensed for systemic use in reversing serious infections such as encephalitis, but licensing seems to be imminent. It has been used quite effectively for these purposes in research centers.

Topically, ACG can also be used against eye infections.

- **Adenine arabinoside** (ara A or Vidarabine) has many of the same properties as ACG, but has been licensed for systemic use. Until ACG *is* licensed, ara A will be the drug of choice for systemic use.
- **2-Deoxy-D-Glucose** (2DG) is used topically, in the treatment of skin lesions, but like ACG and ara A is of limited (and possibly no) use against recurrent infection, although it *may* shorten the length of the attack, and *may* relieve some of its symptoms. Like the others, it is most effective against primary infection, but *unlike* them does not interfere with the genetic mechanics of a normal cell.

  2DG is currently available only through research centers.
- **Interferon** is useful for eye infections, but has not been found to be effective for skin lesions or serious systemic infections due to HSV.

OTHER TREATMENTS FOR HSV-1 AND HSV-2 INFECTIONS

Some previously used treatments which were *not found to be effective* in randomized clinical studies (and which may even in some cases be harmful) *are:*

- smallpox vaccine
- levamisole
- yellow dye/fluorescent light therapy
- ether applications

There has also been a series of vaccines developed to control HSV infection, but while this first generation of vaccines has not proved useful (one of the reasons is the many different strains of HSV), this is an area of active and well-financed research. Improved vaccine technology *has* led to an effective vaccine for varicella zoster (chicken pox and shingles) and shows promise in leading the way to the development of vaccines for HSV.

"MANAGEMENT" OF HSV

It is important to understand that no antiviral—and indeed no other treatment of any kind—has been *demonstrated* to reduce the incidence of recurrence of HSV-1 and HSV-2. Obviously, *avoiding* factors which may *precipitate* an attack of HSV is a wise and conservative approach, and may bring relief to the herpes sufferer. Because of the probable emotional component of the syndrome of recurrent HSV, therefore, stress reduction—and by implication, whatever you *think* works (clinically known as the placebo effect)—can't hurt and may be of significant help.

Although there are no controlled clinical studies that indicate its efficacy, stress reduction—whether through chemotherapy (prescription drugs like tranquilizers), psychotherapy, meditation, biofeedback or imaging—appears to be the most useful (and in fact the most direct) intervention for many people who have HSV.

THE NATUROPATHIC ROUTE

There is absolutely no evidence in randomized clinical studies that either special diets or vitamins help in the management of HSV; all data are purely anecdotal and are useful to the extent of a placebo-effect explanation. However, a change of diet—or a *judicious* vitamin regimen—is unlikely to *hurt* you. Here is what the nature-lovers suggest:

- diets high in L-lysine—which they claim inhibits HSV replication—and low in arginine—which promotes it. L-lysine is an amino acid found in dairy foods, meat, fish, and beans, and is available in pure form—as a dietary supplement—in health-food stores. Arginine, another amino acid, is found in whole grains, chocolate, seeds, nuts, and raisins.
- vitamin C, long attributed by some sectors with a significant role in the effective functioning of the immune system. We *do* know that the status of the immune system is a factor in HSV recurrences.

RELIEVING THE SYMPTOMS OF HSV

People will use just about anything to get relief from the pain and itching of an HSV lesion; the popular literature is full of suggestions, from reasonable to bizarre. You should remember, once again, that the placebo effect appears to be especially powerful in the case of HSV. This doesn't mean that you shouldn't use something to get relief that *brings* you relief (as long as it does no harm), but it does mean that there are no surefire symptom alleviators.

The main thing is to <u>speed healing by keeping the lesion clean and dry.</u> (One of the major drawbacks to the use of the topical antivirals in their present form—cream or ointment—is that they keep the lesion moist.) <u>Astringents and oxidants</u> like alcohol, witch hazel, and Clorox (yes, the laundry bleach) <u>may accomplish this.</u> Agents that do not contribute to the drying process because of their ointment form, but do bring <u>temporary local relief</u> are <u>topical anesthetics</u> such as Xylocaine and lidocaine. Ice packs may help swelling and discomfort. (See following section for particulars.)

THE ALL-CLEAR SIGNAL

The shedding of virus—except in a *small* percentage of cases—stops with the *complete* healing of open sores. In other words, when HSV *looks* like it's gone, and *feels* like it's gone, it's gone. And you and your partner are likely to be safe to have whatever contact you wish without fear of transmitting the infection.

SPECIAL CONSIDERATIONS

Herpesviruses are a threat to any immunologically compromised individual, including the fetus, the newborn, people who are already sick or malnourished, and those who take immunosuppressant drugs (e.g., chemotherapy for a malignancy) or have congenital or acquired immune deficiency diseases.

For these people, HSV may develop into a serious disease (see the earlier discussion of complications) that can be life-threatening.

See HSV-1 and HSV-2 sections for Special Considerations information pertinent to each of these infections.

HELP FOR THE HERPES SUFFERER

HSV victims have their own information clearing house and hotline: the **Herpes Resource Center.** The Center publishes a quarterly newsletter, *The Helper* (which a $12 membership fee entitles you to receive), and is the central office and referral source for forty-five HELP chapters around the country that offer information and group support to their 30,000 members.

You can try contacting the HELP chapter in your area directly, but because of the sensitivity and desire for confidentiality of some members, many of the groups are still underground. The Herpes Resource Center will be glad to put you in touch with your chapter, refer you to a doctor if necessary . . . or just talk with you if you want.

Its mailing address is

Herpes Resource Center
P.O. Box 100
Palo Alto, CA 94302

Its street address is

260 Sheridan Avenue
Suite 307
Palo Alto, CA 94302

Its telephone number is

415-328-7710

These are nice people, who understand your problem (in fact, they usually share it), and are armed with the latest information about HSV. If you want to know more about HSV, get in touch with them.

HSV-1/Oral Herpes Simplex Virus

commonly associated with lesions on the mouth and lips:
cold sores and fever blisters

THINGS YOU NEED TO KNOW

- All generalities about HSV (see preceding section) apply to HSV-1, including its unrestricted "geography," although it most frequently occurs on the lips and is usually passed by mouth-to-mouth contact . . . meaning that strictly speaking, it is not a sexual infection although it can appear on the genitals.
- Most people are exposed to—and contract—HSV-1 before they are 5 years old. 95% of us have antibodies to the virus—indicating previous infection—by the time we are 17 years old.
- The primary infection is inside the mouth, or sometimes on the lips. Subsequent infections are on the outside of the lips, in the cracks at the corners of the mouth, or in the fold at the base of the nostril. Recurrent lesions inside the mouth are rarely herpetic in nature, but rather represent what are called *apthous ulcers* or canker sores, about which little is known.
- Probably half of all people will never have a secondary infection; the virus will remain dormant all their lives. **Only 5– 10% of those infected will ever be troubled by frequent recurrences.**
- Physical factors which predispose people to recurrences are shaving, sunburn (or even exposure to sunlight), menstruation, pregnancy, mouth irritation or trauma (such as biting your lip), and illness/fever. Emotional stress may also be a frequent trigger of HSV-1.
- **Oral HSV is rarely more than a nuisance** . . . and cosmetically unattractive.

WHERE YOU CATCH IT
AND HOW YOU CATCH IT

most frequently <u>on and around the mouth,</u> with the primary lesion inside the mouth. However, any skin surface that comes into <u>contact</u> with an active lesion or infected saliva is vulnerable to invasion—the nipple, for instance. HSV-1 can also be transmitted to the genitals by oral-genital contact, or to the eyes by the hands or saliva.

SIGNS AND SYMPTOMS

- **Primary infection** appears in <u>3–5 days,</u> with fever, lymph node enlargement in the neck, and the development of multiple small ulcers on the inside surface of the mouth, on the tongue, and around the teeth. The pain associated with a primary attack may interfere with eating and drinking, particularly in small children, and lead to dehydration.
- **Secondary infection** usually <u>occurs on the outer borders of the lips,</u> but may attack any skin surface served by the infected sensory nerve, including the face and even the eye (herpes keratitis; see discussion below of complications). A blister—or a small group of blisters—will form, break, crust over, and scab.

    Secondary infections often announce themselves with a tingling or aching before the blisters appear (prodrome) or a general sensation of low-grade fever or flu.

    <u>HSV-1 is considered to be infectious from the inception of the prodrome.</u>

COMPLICATIONS

- **herpes keratitis**—either when the eye is contaminated by infected saliva, or when the nerve bundle serving the original site, which also serves the eye, is infected
- **encephalitis**—when the virus infects the brain. *Herpes encephalitis is very rare* and can lead to death or serious brain damage.

- **secondary bacterial infection**—when bacteria enter the open lesion, with the usual complications of a bacterial infection: swelling, inflammation, and pus

DIAGNOSIS

- inspection
- culture

See discussion of diagnosis in earlier section, Herpesviruses—In General.

TREATMENT

Topical treatment with new antivirals may shorten the duration of cold sores, but they cannot cure the infection in the nerve cell, where it remains dormant.

In terms of symptom relief, there is always the conflict between keeping the lesion moist to prevent cracking of the lips or corners of the mouth (which tends to prolong healing) or keeping it dry (which tends to promote it). Agents made for dry or sunburned lips may make you feel more comfortable, but be sure to use something that is not applied directly to the mouth—like a lipstick—but is rather an ointment-type preparation that you will not contaminate during use.

THE ALL-CLEAR SIGNAL

When the lesions have disappeared, you can usually consider yourself noninfective.

While a small minority of HSV-1 sufferers continue to excrete low concentrations of virus in the saliva in the absence of identifiable lesions, it is thought unlikely that these levels can transmit infection. You need not, therefore, be concerned that your saliva is swarming with organisms when you are not in the active phase.

Dentists—who should be most worried about asymptomatic shedding of HSV in the saliva—are, for the most part, thoroughly unperturbed by the current flap. The fact is that dentists *do* get finger lesions occasionally, but like most people they resist recurrences.

Some dentists routinely ask patients whether they have recurrences of HSV-1; if your dentist *doesn't* ask, and you *do* have *recurrent cold sores* (*not* genital herpes), be sure to inform him, as it is part of your dental health profile. You are unlikely, at any rate, to want to go for dental work if you are in the active phase.

Once again, *genital* herpes does not render your *saliva* infectious; *oral* herpes does not make *genital* secretions infectious. This is *not* a systemic disease (except in the rarest cases).

SPECIAL CONSIDERATIONS ABOUT NEWBORNS

While most HSV infections of the newborn are of Type II and transmitted during vaginal delivery, infection from oral lesions has been recorded. HSV transmitted by oral secretions to a new baby carries the same grave—and potentially fatal—consequences as does HSV infection picked up from a mother infected with active genital herpes at the time of delivery.

In other words, **don't let Aunt Gertie kiss the baby if she has a cold sore.**

HSV-2/Genital Herpes Simplex Virus

commonly associated with lesions on the genitals, and on the cervix in women

THINGS YOU NEED TO KNOW

- All generalities about HSV (see earlier section, Herpesviruses—In General) apply to HSV-2—including its unrestricted "geography," although HSV-2 most frequently occurs on the genitals, buttocks, or thighs.
- HSV-2 is currently considered to be epidemic. It is not unlikely, however, that this "exponential rise" in the occurrence of the infection is less directly attributable to its virulence than to its enormously increased visibility and to

the attention given it by the media and the medical profession. While recent epidemiological studies indicate that approximately twenty million Americans have HSV-2 (this translates to one out of five adults) with another half a million added annually, the longer-term observation that in many segments of the population, over 60% of people have antibodies to HSV-2—indicating previous (probably subclinical) infection—by the age of 21 is perhaps even more interesting.

- **There is no reason for HSV-2 to ruin your life.** Current media overkill about herpes is worse than misleading . . . it's brutally irresponsible. So what if herpes is incurable? So is chicken pox. So what if you may be one of the few in whom it recurs? You're much more likely—as are the people you know—to get recurrences of varicella zoster (chickenpox) in the form of shingles when you are older. And when was the last time you heard about somebody traumatized by shingles? Or a cold sore?

  Genital herpes should be nothing more than a minor annoyance, with *no* implications for someone who is not pregnant, newborn, or immunologically compromised. (See Herpesviruses—In General and The "Terrible Curse" of Herpes.) **Having HSV-2 should not destroy your sense of self-esteem nor interfere with any more of your life than simple prudence would dictate:** it makes no more sense to have sex if you or your partner has active HSV-2 than it does to kiss if either of you has active HSV-1. **Having herpes has *nothing* to do with your "moral" character.**

  The only other realistic concern about HSV-2 has to do with its potential linkage to cervical cancer in women (see Special Cautions). Frequent Pap smears and careful observation by your gynecologist will lead to early detection—and proper treatment—of any cervical changes.

- **More than half the people who have HSV-2 will never have another attack after the first one. Only 5–10% of those infected will be real sufferers,** with recurrences that are sometimes as frequent as once a month. The rest of the people with HSV-2 fall in between, with an occasional flare-up that usually occurs less than once a year.

- Factors which predispose people to recurrences of genital herpes are local irritations—like the rubbing of clothes, bodies, or genitals; menstruation, pregnancy, or birth-control pills; heat or being run-down.

Emotional stress and anxiety, however, are probably responsible for more recurrences than all the other factors put together. This is the way in which HSV-2 feeds on and perpetuates itself.

- HSV-2 does not ping-pong as do many other sexual infections. Once you've got it, you've got it, and in almost all cases recurrences are of latent infection, rather than a symptom of a new one.

Technically, because there are many strains of HSV-2, it is *possible* to be infected with another strain, although for all practical purposes this should not be of concern to the average person. The fact that reinfection *can* occur is more relevant to theoretical considerations of the nature of the course of infection, and to scientists in their attempts to develop a vaccine.

- **Those people who suffer from frequent recurrences of HSV-2 have not been shown to differ from infected people who *do not* have recurrences in either their sexual practices, number of partners, or frequency of their sexual contacts.** In other words, there is no social or moral significance —one way or the other—to the rate at which you are susceptible to attacks.

WHERE YOU CATCH IT AND HOW YOU CATCH IT

HSV-2 is usually found below the waist—especially on the genitals, although it may also appear on buttocks, thighs, or calves. It can be transmitted to the mouth during oral sex.

Any skin surface that comes into contact with an active lesion or infected secretions is vulnerable to invasion. Some experts consider recurrent HSV to be communicable from the first signs of the **prodrome.**

SIGNS AND SYMPTOMS

- **Primary infection** appears in 2–20 days (average: 6), often with fever, aching muscles, and swollen glands in the groin (and sometimes elsewhere). You can feel quite ill with a primary attack.

When the blisters appear, they are usually accompanied by local swelling (some women may have painful engorgement of the clitoris and labia), itching, and possibly burning—particularly if lesions get wet when you urinate.

Primary attacks may take as long as two or three weeks to dissipate. It is essential to see a doctor—even if you think you know what you have—not only because there are other blisterlike and/or ulcerated sores that may be mistaken for HSV-2 and be something else that is more dangerous (like a syphilis chancre), but because some of the new antivirals seem to be topically effective only in primary attacks . . . and then only when they are used early.

- **Secondary infections** are almost always less severe—and less long-lasting—than primaries. It is still not clear why many people *never* have a recurrence, and a few people have many, but it is undoubtedly related to general health—emotional as well as physical—and the strength of a person's resistance, which can be both environmentally and genetically determined.

Recurrences often announce themselves with a **prodrome:** itching, tingling, aching, or burning sensations that can either be restricted to the immediate area of the eventual outbreak, or may affect a much larger portion of the body. (Sometimes the sensations affect the whole lower quadrant in which the nerves that serve the original site are located, as if there were two lines drawn—one around the waist, and one bisecting the body, through the genitals, from the waist in front to the waist in back. This is a result of the bilateral characteristics of the nervous system, and irritation of adjacent nerve bundles.) The burning sensation of the prodrome—topical skin sensitivity—is a feeling not unlike sunburn; the aching of the prodrome can feel bone-deep and sometimes makes it difficult to walk.

The prodrome tends to fade as the sores develop.

The course of a secondary infection runs anywhere from 5 to 10 days.

COMPLICATIONS

- **secondary bacterial infection** when bacteria invade the open sores, with the usual complications of bacterial infection: swelling, inflammation, and pus, possible lymph node involvement
- (very rarely) **spinal meningitis,** when the virus attacks the spinal cord
- **cancer of the cervix** in women has been associated with HSV-2, although no *causal* connection has been made. The facts are:

  a) A large proportion of patients with diagnosed cervical cancer have antibodies to HSV-2.
  b) One quarter of the women who have recurrent HSV-2 show—over time—cervical changes consistent with pre-malignant states.
  c) A woman with recurrent HSV-2 has a five to ten times greater risk of developing cervical cancer.

  However, careful gynecological follow-up with Pap smears every six to twelve months is good insurance against such pre-cancerous conditions, which can be controlled with considerable success.
- **infection of the newborn** by transmission of the virus from active genital lesions at the time of vaginal delivery. This frequently has tragic consequences. See Special Considerations.

DIAGNOSIS

- inspection. Although HSV-2 has a characteristic presentation, it is too frequently misdiagnosed. The only way to be *sure* that a lesion is herpetic is by
- culture. See the earlier section, Herpesviruses—In General.
- blood test. Evidence of development—or rising titre—of specific antibodies.

TREATMENT

There is no treatment for HSV-2 that has been demonstrated to be effective. This includes the new antivirals (which *may* help somewhat in primary attacks, and *may* shorten the length of the attack or the period of viral shedding) or any one of dozens of treatments that have been tried and discarded over the years.

It is important to keep the sores clean and dry to prevent secondary infection, and not to irritate them by wearing tight clothing that rubs or doesn't "breathe" (this includes jockey shorts, elastic-leg panties, and pantyhose). Warm baths are soothing, and you can use *Epsom salts, baking soda,* or *Burrow's solution* to stay clean and relieve discomfort. Some people use local anesthetic ointments to alleviate pain . . . which can be so intense, especially during urination, that urinary retention becomes a serious problem; their drawback is their lack of drying properties. (If you *are* having trouble urinating—this usually happens only during a primary attack—try running a bathtub full of water, getting in, and *then* urinating. It's better than having to be catheterized.)

Agents that promote drying—and have oxidizing properties— seem to speed healing. A few such agents are Clorox (the laundry bleach), alcohol, witch hazel, and ketone. Apply these with a Q-tip directly to the sore.

Because of the emotional component of HSV-2, it is helpful and reassuring to remember that whatever seems to work for you either in alleviating the symptoms of an attack, or in heading off a state of mind which seems to welcome a recurrence—*and* causes no damage—is "effective" treatment in the absence of a cure.

A last note: sometimes HSV-2 sufferers fantasize about somehow cutting off or cutting out the piece of tissue that continually succumbs to the sores or blisters. The virus lives in the nerve fibers, however, and can't be cut out of *them,* so it would simply find a new outlet to the surface of the skin. The problem is *in* you, not *on* you.

THE ALL-CLEAR SIGNAL

When the sores are gone, and the scabs have fallen off, you can usually consider yourself no longer infectious, especially if you are male (which means that any and all lesions are *visible*).

If you are female, knowing when you do—and when you do not—have active lesions is not quite so simple. Medical researchers are not yet sure how frequently cervical and vulvar lesions co-occur—that is, whether a woman who has vulvar recurrences can have an active cervical infection (which is usually asymptomatic) *without* vulvar manifestation. This means that if a woman has vulvar lesions she *will* know when she is infectious, and if she has cervical lesions *alone,* she may *not.* Furthermore, any woman who has cervical lesions—with or without accompanying sores on the vulva—may at some time show a positive cervical culture *between* attacks . . . although it is generally thought that viral concentrations at such times are too low to communicate the infection. Indeed, empirical observation strongly suggests that women with recurrent HSV-2 can have very active sex lives and *never* infect a partner . . . *if* they stay alert to signs of imminent attack or the active phase.

Male partners who are concerned about exposure to asymptomatic cervical lesions, or women who are concerned for their partners, can use condoms or diaphragms, which provide at least partial protection.

P.S.: Stay in touch with the Herpes Resource Center for developments.

SPECIAL CONSIDERATIONS FOR WOMEN

- Women with recurrent HSV-2 should have regular Pap smears to monitor cervical changes that can be early indicators of malignancy. (See HSV-2 Complications above.)
- HSV-2 infections are frequently associated with both *Hemophilus vaginalis* and *Trichomoniasis* (the relationship to trich is particularly close and not yet fully understood). You should be checked regularly for both these infections if you have HSV-2.
- HSV-2 has been linked to cancer of the vulva.

SPECIAL CONSIDERATIONS FOR PREGNANT WOMEN

Infecting your baby with HSV-2 can kill him/her or cause brain damage: about half the women with *active lesions at the time of vaginal delivery* will infect their infants, about 60% of the babies who catch it will die, and half the survivors will be blind or brain-damaged.

Most of the women who infect their babies, however, do not know they have HSV-2. Women who are aware of their infections can protect themselves and their newborns by having cultures throughout pregnancy, and every week for the last month of gestation.

If herpesvirus is found in the final 4 weeks of pregnancy, or if active infection is present—whether it is cultured or not—a Caesarean section is usually planned on. Immediate emergency C-sections are also done if the water breaks while the mother has an active infection, as the virus can ascend the birth canal within hours.

You must always tell your obstetrician—and be monitored by him/ her—during your pregnancy if you are an HSV-2 sufferer.

PROTECTING YOURSELF FROM GENITAL HERPES

Barrier methods of contraception are considered to be at least partially effective protection if you are concerned about contracting—or spreading—HSV-2 infection either during periods of perceived inactivity or in cases where active periods are difficult to demarcate because of lack of symptoms. Also, some spermicides used with diaphragms and in foam have been found to be viricidal to HSV in tissue culture.

It should go without saying that there ought to be *no* sexual contact if either you or a partner with HSV-2 is in the *active* phase.

Cytomegalovirus (CMV)

a systemic infection caused by a virus (CMV) in the herpesvirus family

THINGS YOU NEED TO KNOW

- CMV infections are very common. About 80% of adults over 40 have antibodies to this virus, which means that they have at some time been exposed to CMV.

- In most people, CMV infections have no symptoms . . . and cause no problems. Some people may develop mononucleosis or a mononucleosis-like disease.
- CMV infects the unborn infant and may cause death, severe mental retardation, or birth defects.
- CMV can cause lethal pneumonia and hepatitis in people with reduced resistance, i.e., people with chronic disease or malignancies, or certain homosexuals.
- CMV can be transmitted in saliva, sexual secretions, or blood transfusions.

WHERE YOU CATCH IT

Women	cervix
	urethra
Men	urethra
	prostate
Both	salivary glands

HOW YOU CATCH IT

- contact with infected oral or genital secretions, in any combination: kissing, oral sex, coitus
- blood transfusions

SYMPTOMS

CMV rarely has symptoms in otherwise healthy people; prior infection is surmised by the presence of antibodies in the blood. Occasionally such people will develop a mononucleosis-like disease.

Symptoms are more serious in those people whose immunity is compromised by (1) immaturity, as in the fetus; (2) drugs like those used in cancer chemotherapy; (3) hormones, such as those produced during pregnancy; or (4) other infections.

WHAT IT DOES

CMV initially infects local tissues, in particular the salivary glands, the prostate, and the cervix. It then invades the bloodstream, where it can be carried by certain white cells and transmitted to other tissues such as the liver, spleen, kidneys, lungs, and lymph nodes, causing secondary infections and the destruction of cells within these organs. This process is what causes the symptoms of mononucleosis: fever, swollen glands, enlargement of the liver and spleen, weakness and fatigue, muscle and joint aches, and a general feeling of illness. Hepatitis and jaundice may also develop.

DIAGNOSIS

- by **culturing** the virus from infected secretions (saliva, semen, vaginal secretions, urine, or blood), or
- by documentation of a rapid and significant rise of the antibody in the blood (by **blood test**)

TREATMENT

As is true for most viruses, no effective treatment has been established. New anti-viral drugs are currently being tested in university centers.

CMV, like other infections of the herpesvirus family, can remain latent in the body for extended periods of time before being activated for reasons usually having to do with lowered resistance to infection.

THE ALL-CLEAR SIGNAL

Active infection is considered to be at an end when the virus can no longer be cultured from the urine, blood, or other secretions. The duration of active infection—with virus excretion—is variable; it may last for years.

SPECIAL CONSIDERATIONS FOR PREGNANT WOMEN

CMV may be passed to the fetus across the placenta early in pregnancy. **The fetus has little or no resistance to this virus, which causes severe damage** to the brain, eyes, ears, liver, and lungs—producing mental retardation, blindness, deafness, hepatitis, pneumonia . . . and a significant rate of fetal death. One quarter of all serious mental retardation in infants is caused by CMV.

Breast milk may also contain virus if the mother has an active infection.

SPECIAL CONSIDERATION FOR HOMOSEXUAL MEN

For some as yet undetermined reason, certain homosexuals are susceptible to CMV. Their infections may be associated with severe hepatitis and pneumonia.

In Africa, CMV has been linked to a malignancy called Kaposi's sarcoma. **Whether this connection also holds true for the Kaposi's sarcoma increasingly reported in homosexual men who are also infected with CMV is not known, but no *causal* relationship has been established.**

SPECIAL CONSIDERATIONS FOR PEOPLE WITH IMMUNE DEFICIENCIES

People who are receiving immunosuppresant drugs—cancer patients undergoing chemotherapy would be one example—should be aware of their high-risk status for CMV.

Epstein-Barr Virus (EBV)

a DNA virus in the herpesvirus group which causes most
of the cases of infectious mononucleosis

THINGS YOU NEED TO KNOW

- EBV infections are very common (85% of children are infected before they are 15) but rarely symptomatic.
- EBV infections usually clear up by themselves, although active virus may be detected in blood cells for a long period of time. (Latent virus—as with any herpesvirus infection—may always be in the body.) Antibodies specific to EBV will also be produced for many years following active infection.
- EBV is frequently identified with infectious mononucleosis and its more acute symptoms, but low-grade chronic infections may be manifested by a vague feeling of illness and fatigue that can last for months . . . or years.
- Of all the herpesviruses, the link between EBV and cancer is the strongest. It has been implicated in a cancer called Burkitt's lymphoma (usually seen in Africa), in a nose-and-throat

cancer among the Chinese, and in certain lymphatic disorders—that *may* be malignant—observed in congenitally immune-deficient children and in immune-suppressed patients like people who have cancer, and transplant (particularly kidney) recipients.

- It is believed, therefore, that an effective immune response is needed to keep EBV—which most of us "have"—in check. Reactivation of latent infection occurs when the resistance of a person is somehow impaired.

HOW YOU CATCH IT

Although the virus is most frequently passed by mouth (which is why infectious mononucleosis is sometimes called "the kissing disease"), recent evidence suggests that it can be transmitted through sexual contact by sexual secretions from someone who has an active infection.

EBV can also be transmitted through blood transfusions.

SYMPTOMS

Infectious mononucleosis (the clinical expression of EBV, especially in young people) is a long-lasting infection with a rapid onset of symptoms: malaise, sore throat, and enlargement of lymph nodes—particularly in the neck (draining the mouth as the primary site of infection) and the spleen. The fatigue and malaise may last a long time, and EBV may also cause hepatitis, which is most often mild but can be serious. Other symptoms may include an inflammation of small blood vessels (thereby giving rise to characteristic skin rashes), abdominal pain from inflamed and swollen tissue membranes like the peritoneum, or swelling, pain and stiffness in the joints from the inflammation of the fluid-producing membranes which cushion them.

WHAT IT DOES

The virus is principally passed in salivary secretions but may also be transmitted in genital secretions. Following infection of local tissues—such as the throat—the virus rapidly spreads to lymph nodes and the blood system via infection of circulating white cells—particularly certain types of immune cells called B-lymphocytes (a characteristic of which is their capacity to multiply without apparent stimulus). Development of these lymphocytes in the spleen and lymph nodes—and the generation of other types of immune lymphocytes *toxic* to these infected cells—results in enlargement of affected tissues. (The large numbers of activated or "atypical" lymphocytes detected in the blood are predominantly the immune cells capable of killing those that are virus-infected.)

EBV may infect secretory tissues such as the salivary glands and accessory genital glands and may also infect the liver. It is likely that abnormalities in function of these organs is more readily attributable to the immune response than to the virus itself (see above).

For the vast majority of people, however, EBV infections are totally asymptomatic and rarely cause clinically significant disease.

DIAGNOSIS

a **typical clinical picture** (to your doctor), **accompanied by** an increase in atypical lymphocytes in the blood and a clear rise in characteristic antibodies (determined by **blood test)**

TREATMENT

No agent has yet been shown to be effective in controlling severe infections. Fortunately, such infections are rare. With rest and the tincture of time, the body achieves its own control of infection, and clinical symptoms slowly resolve.

In short, EBV "goes away"—which is really a retreat to the *subclinical* phase—by itself.

SPECIAL CONSIDERATIONS FOR PREGNANT WOMEN

Rare case reports suggest that EBV from an *actively* infected mother can be transferred across the placenta to the fetus, leading to congenital abnormalities, blood-cell disorders, and neurological damage.

SPECIAL CONSIDERATIONS FOR HOMOSEXUAL MEN

For some reason having to do with not-yet-understood and poorly defined immune deficiencies, certain homosexual men experience reactivation of the virus and occurrence of clinically significant infections (see discussion of AIDS in For Gay Men, Part III).

SPECIAL CONSIDERATIONS FOR PEOPLE WITH IMMUNE DEFICIENCIES

People with special types of deficiencies—certain of which are genetic, others of which are presumably chemically induced—are at a much higher risk for severe EBV infection.

Other Viral Infections

Venereal Warts

Non-malignant skin growths occurring in a number of forms (most frequently as *condylomata accuminata*) caused by certain types of human papillomaviruses (HPV)

THINGS YOU NEED TO KNOW

- Venereal warts occur in many forms and may be caused by a number of different papillomaviruses. The most common kind is one that grows in little cauliflowerlike clusters— hence the name condylomata accuminata. Venereal warts are not caused by the same viruses as those that are responsible for warts on the hands or on the feet.
- Venereal warts are only transmitted sexually (except in the rarest of cases), and they are highly contagious. Up to 80% of people having regular contact with a partner who has warts will catch them.
- Warts have an unusually long incubation period, taking anywhere from 6 weeks to 6 months to appear after having been caught. (The average time is 2–3 months.) Warts are contagious during the incubation period, that is, before they appear.
- Wart growth is closely tied to fluctuations in someone's resistance. Or their hormone levels. (Pregnant women are particularly susceptible.)

- In women, warts are frequently associated with other sexual infections, particularly gonorrhea and trichomoniasis.
- The second most frequently observed venereal wart is called a *flat condyloma.* It may appear on other parts of the body, and must be seen by a doctor (and usually biopsied) to be distinguished from the wide flat growths, called condylomata lata, of syphilis. Flat warts suggest a possible association with cervical cancer in women.
- Venereal warts usually do not go away by themselves. If they are not treated, they are likely to multiply and make treatment even more difficult.
- Venereal warts frequently recur, probably as a result of reinfection. For this reason, any partner should also be checked by a doctor for warts.
- Warts can be hidden (and often are) in the vagina or anus.

WHERE YOU CATCH THEM

Women vulva
labia
vagina
cervix
perineum (frequently)
Men penis (especially if uncircumcised)
urethra
bladder
Both anus (from rectal coitus)
mouth (rare)
throat (rare)

Warts like wet surfaces and skin folds (where they often spread to the facing surface) such as between the labia, under the foreskin, on the perineum, and between the buttocks.

HOW YOU CATCH THEM

sexual contact or contact of irritated tissues with a wart. Venereal warts are highly contagious.

SYMPTOMS

usually take from **2 to 3 months** to develop. Venereal warts begin as small round red painless bumps. They may be single, but usually come in groups. As they enlarge, they frequently begin to look like little fleshy cauliflowers, although the growths can take many forms.

WHAT THEY DO

The virus induces growths in the surface of the infected skin and adjacent mucous membranes. They spread easily and may quickly infect surrounding tissue.

Frequently wart growth and spread fluctuates as a function of the resources of the immune system (people on immunosuppressant drugs and steroids are particularly susceptible) and hormonal levels (pregnant women and those taking birth-control pills are susceptible).

For reasons not yet well understood, spontaneous resolution of warts is not unusual. Because they are unattractive and bothersome, however, and because they are more likely to get worse than get better, people usually choose to have them removed.

DIAGNOSIS

- clinical **examination**
- **biopsy** (to rule out malignancies, especially if the wart is painful, oozing, or chronically abraded)
- **immunofluorescence tests:** new techniques measuring the reaction of papillomavirus-specific antibodies, permitting accurate detection of virus in affected tissues

TREATMENT

Unlike the herpesviruses, venereal warts can be treated with agents that kill the affected tissues, warts and all:
- podophyllin—a chemical—is the most frequently used agent against warts because it is quick and easy . . . although it must be carefully monitored: It has to be washed off about 3 hours after treatment or it can cause painful burns. Furthermore, its absorption by the body over longer periods could result in neurological damage and the depression of blood formation.

Podophyllin also changes some of the normal characteristics of the tissues, so that a later biopsy of a podophyllin-treated lesion may be difficult—if not impossible—to interpret.

Pregnant women—for the reasons cited above about systemic effects—**should never have warts—*any* warts—removed with podophyllin.**

- <u>burning or cauterization</u>—either by chemical means (acid) or by surgical cautery
- <u>freezing</u> (cryosurgery)—either with CO_2 snow or with liquid nitrogen
- <u>surgical excision</u>

All of the above methods are effective. Two drawbacks they share are (1) that treatment can be fairly uncomfortable (your doctor may use a local anesthetic to alleviate pain) and (2) they leave scars. Scarring can at some later time lead to obstructions (if, for example, it is in the anus or urethra) that may then need to be corrected surgically.

There is one new method that leaves minimal scar tissue:

- carbon dioxide <u>laser beams,</u> usually found only in hospitals, and requiring highly skilled handling. Laser treatment can destroy the entire infected cell as effectively as the other methods without their attendant disadvantages; it can usually be done without anesthesia, and there is minimal scarring.

THE ALL-CLEAR SIGNAL

When the lesions have scarred over, they are considered to be healed.

SPECIAL CONSIDERATIONS FOR WOMEN

- Venereal warts often coexist in women with other sexual infections, particularly gonorrhea and trichomoniasis. Make sure that you are checked for these infections if warts are diagnosed.
- Warts may be hidden deep in the vagina or on the cervix, where they can cause considerable degeneration before they are diagnosed. Furthermore, advanced infection with venereal warts can cause tissue changes that are consistent with pre-malignant disorders (carcinoma *in situ*). The good news is that these changes are easily

detectable in Pap smears . . . just one more reason to make sure Pap smears are a regular part of your gynecological checkup.
- Birth-control pills and pregnancy stimulate the growth and spread of venereal warts.

SPECIAL CONSIDERATIONS FOR PREGNANT WOMEN

While venereal warts do not affect the unborn child, they *can* be picked up during vaginal delivery by the newborn, infecting its throat. Laryngeal warts may lead to obstructed breathing in babies that are severely affected, and to hoarseness and difficulty in speaking in older children and adults.

SPECIAL CONSIDERATIONS FOR MEN

Some men have *penile papules*—pearly bumps that may look like little warts but are not. These come from enlargement of sebaceous glands, particularly around the head of the penis, and are normal. (The clinical picture can be confusing, but biopsy will show normal tissue.)

Molluscum Contagiosum

a mildly contagious skin condition caused by a human poxvirus

THINGS YOU NEED TO KNOW

- Molluscum is not, strictly speaking, a sexual infection because it can be picked up in many kinds of close physical contact, including swimming pools and locker rooms. It is in this book because it can also be sexually transmitted—when it occurs almost exclusively around the genitals, thighs, and buttocks—and is turning up with increasing frequency in venereal-disease and public-health facilities. If you happen to get it, you should know what it is.
- Molluscum is characterized by small hard whitish or yellowish bumps that tend to occur in multiples. A distinguishing

characteristic is a central depression (a sort of dimple) in the middle of each bump.

- Molluscum doesn't hurt and has no other symptoms. It *may* go away by itself.
- The infection grows and progresses slowly, usually over a period of many months.

WHERE YOU GET IT

genitals
buttocks (especially in homosexual men)
thighs
abdomen

HOW YOU GET IT

- sexual or other intimate bodily contact
- from a warm wet surface that can briefly sustain the viability of the organism

SYMPTOMS

Lesions may appear any time from **3 weeks to 3 months** after exposure. There are usually no other symptoms (occasionally the bumps may itch) unless there is secondary infection.

WHAT IT DOES

Molluscum makes itself a capsule as it invades the skin surface, and once established, causes degeneration of skin cells and compresses the connective tissue in deeper levels of skin.

DIAGNOSIS

by **inspection**

TREATMENT

Molluscum lesions can be scraped off with a curette (a surgeon's knife), or punctured and squeezed. There is a hard white grain inside. Sometimes medication to inhibit recurrence is applied.

THE ALL-CLEAR SIGNAL

When the bumps—and their contents—have been scraped off, the infection is gone.

FUNGUS INFECTIONS

candidiasis (formerly called monilia or moniliasis) • *tinea cruris (jock itch)*

FUNGUSES
  are free-living, microscopic, plantlike organisms that live in and off moist, decaying organic matter. There are about 100 funguses that cause human disease, and of these, only *candida* and the *dermatophytes* (which include skin conditions like jock itch and athlete's foot) are transmitted from person to person.

These contagious infections are "superficial" infections that—while often chronic (they seem to go away and then come back again) and hard to cure—rarely affect someone's general health. They use the thin, dead (keratinized) surface layer of skin—and the inflammatory response to invasion—as a kind of human culture medium in which to implant, live, and grow.

Funguses are treated topically with fungicides.

Candidiasis
(sometimes known as MONILIA, or MONILIASIS)

a common infection of the skin and mucous membranes caused by a kind of fungal organism called a yeast (yeasts replicate by budding) of the *Candida* family (usually *Candida albicans*)

THINGS YOU NEED TO KNOW

- The organism that causes candidiasis (often referred to as just "candida") is a normal and natural constituent of the vaginal flora that is usually kept in check by competing bacterial organisms. When the vaginal ecology is upset (for instance, when you take antibiotics), candida can overgrow to cause infection. Therefore, it is not *necessarily* sexually transmitted.

- *However,* candida can also be sexually transmitted, although the organism rarely outgrows the skin bacteria on the male genitals to cause an obvious infection. Candida does not grow naturally in the urethra, but may cause a urethritis in men. It is more likely to cause a condition called *balanitis* (inflammation of the glans of the penis and the foreskin), which is seen in 10% of the male partners of women who have candidiasis.

- About 20% of all **vaginitis** is caused by candida, and while it is not serious, the itching can drive you crazy. It can also cause damage to the vaginal mucosa, making you susceptible to the invasion of other pathogens.

- A candida overgrowth in the mouth is called **thrush,** and is most frequently seen in newborns who are infected by candida during vaginal delivery. Adults can also develop thrush in response to massive doses of antibiotics, or under certain medical circumstances.

WHERE YOU GET IT AND ITS SYMPTOMS

Women   vagina
- turns bright red
- cheesy-looking, yeasty-smelling discharge (sometimes)

		• white patches (plaques) on cervix and vaginal walls
		• painful intercourse (dyspareunia)
	vulva	• turns red
		• itches like mad, especially at night
		• is dry and tender, with a "thin-skinned" feel
Men	penis	• itching
		• redness
		• inflammation and swelling
Both	urethra	• burning on urination
	mouth (thrush)	• whitish patches on tongue and inside of cheeks
		• sore mouth, tongue, and/or throat, restricting eating and drinking

HOW YOU GET IT

When candida is *not* sexually transmitted, infection in women is a result of a change in normal vaginal microbial ecology. Upsetting of a healthy balance promotes an overgrowth of the organism. Conditions favorable to this overgrowth include:

- anything that changes the level of circulating hormones in a woman's body—birth-control pills, pregnancy, the menstrual cycle.
- taking antibiotics, which kill off the "good" bacteria which protect vaginal health (especially *Lactobacillus*) with the "bad." When the "good" bacteria are depleted, the vagina becomes less acid, and the antibiotic-resistant fungus proliferates rapidly, establishing infection.
- a demonstrable rise in blood sugar level, such as happens in women who are diabetic or pre-diabetic, pregnant, or are being treated with hormones like birth-control pills or steroids (used for the relief of severe allergies, arthritis, or kidney disease).
- wearing clothing that is too tight and/or doesn't "breathe," like panties made of synthetic fibers (rather than natural ones like cotton or silk), pantyhose, and shorts or slacks that are restricting. Synthetics can be abrasive, and don't allow for evaporation of normal vaginal secretions or perspiration.

The combination of irritation and moisture makes an ideal growing medium for candida. The deep skin folds and moist skin associated with being overweight can also increase susceptibility to candida.

WHAT IT DOES

The course of an infection by candida has already been discussed. The itching of candidiasis is caused by hypersensitivity to the chemical constituents and metabolic by-products of the fungus. Inflammation is caused by invasion of the microbe and its capacity to digest outer layers of skin and mucosa, stripping the surface it inhabits.

Unlike bacteria, candida organisms produce no toxins.

DIAGNOSIS

- **wet-mount smear,** done in a doctor's office. The budding yeasts are unusually prominent and readily visible under a microscope. The doctor, however, must determine whether the *presence* of candida indicates responsibility for the vaginitis. Cultures are done to check the concentration of the fungus, or to determine whether a particular site is colonized. *Results:* immediate.
- **culture.** *Results:* 48 hours.

Women should be cultured for gonorrhea at the same time.

In all cases of vaginitis, do not douche before seeing the doctor. It washes away the evidence.

TREATMENT

Candidiasis is one of those conditions for which there are a number of treatments, some of them of the home-remedy variety. *If* **you are sure of what you have** (some women get candida frequently enough to know what it is) **you** *may* **want to self-treat.** *However,* **if there is** *any* **question as to what the infection is— and/or the home remedy proves ineffective—***stop* **the treatment and** *see your doctor.* **There are too many other sexual infections which co-exist with candida to take a chance.**

- by doctor's prescription: various creams and suppositories, the active ingredient of which is an anti-fungal agent such as mycostatin, miconazole, or clotrimazole.

- immediate treatment in the doctor's office . . . and immediate relief: gentian violet, painted on the infected surfaces. *However,* be aware that gentian violet is a chemical dye (with anti-fungal properties) that is a dead ringer for dark-blue ink and it *stains* like ink—clothes, hands, and wherever it is applied. (It fortunately sloughs off and out of the vagina in a few days. Wear a sanitary pad to protect your clothes.)

  If candida is a consistent problem for you—and you think you can manage the painting procedure—your doctor may give you a prescription for the gentian violet and let you treat yourself. *If* you do, you *must* use a *long, sterile* Q-tip, or you will contaminate your bottle of dye. (See For Women in Part III for use of a speculum.)

  Gentian violet is also used for the relief of oral infection by candida.
- boric acid powder, packed (by you, if you choose) into ordinary size 0 (holding 600 mg.) gelatin capsules, and inserted, one per night, into the vagina for a period of 2 weeks. Pricking the capsule with a pin before insertion helps it dissolve faster.

  These capsules are for vaginal use only, and are not to be swallowed.
- yogurt—unflavored, please, and without any of the pudding-like additives—with *live* acidophilus cultures (AKA the friendly *Lactobacillus*—look at the ingredients list). *Eating* yogurt will help to protect *all* your internal ecology (discouraging both candidiasis *and* diarrhea and cramping) when you take antibiotics; *local application* will help restore your *Lactobacillus* balance.

  In addition, yogurt is cheap, available, and very soothing. Just turn yourself upside down (a bathtub is a good place to prop yourself in this position) so that the internal organs fall away from the vaginal opening, and spoon some in. Gravity will do the rest, as long as you stay upside down.
- If you are one of those women who has a good idea when you are vulnerable to overgrowth, you can sometimes nip the yeast in the bud with a vinegar douche (2 tablespoons of white vinegar to a quart of warm water).

THE ALL-CLEAR SIGNAL

You'll know when your yeast infection is gone: the redness and cheesy discharge disappear, and the itching stops.

SPECIAL CONSIDERATIONS FOR WOMEN

- Sometimes women who get candida for the first time jump to conclusions and accuse a partner of having brought an infection into the relationship. Remember that candida is more likely to "develop" than to be "caught."
- Candidiasis can occur because another infection has paved the way for it by upsetting the vaginal ecology. It is always a good idea to be checked for other sexual infections if there is the *slightest* doubt about the reasons for the infection.

SPECIAL CONSIDERATIONS FOR PREGNANT WOMEN

Pregnant women should not be treated with some of the anti-fungal agents. Be sure to check with your doctor before using a standard prescription remedy for candida, and let him/her know that you are pregnant.

Tinea Cruris (Jock Itch)

a fungal infection of the dermatophyte family,
also known as ringworm

THINGS YOU NEED TO KNOW

- Like athlete's foot (another contagious human fungus of the dermatophyte group), jock itch is caught, not "developed." Once caught, it can be very hard to get rid of completely; it can retreat to the subclinical phase often and then recur when conditions are right.
- While jock itch can be transmitted sexually (women get it too) it is also frequently picked up in locker rooms, or from damp towels or clothing that is shared.

- Because <u>jock itch is a chronic infection,</u> a recurrence is likely to have nothing to do with reinfection, but rather with conditions favorable to recolonization by the fungus: like heat, unevaporated perspiration, and abraded skin. (In fact, many of the same conditions which predispose women to candida predispose men to jock itch: tight, nonabsorbent clothing with inadequate ventilation, rubbing, and irritation.)

WHERE YOU CATCH IT

<u>skin</u> of the pubic area (including the testicles) and the upper inner thigh

HOW YOU CATCH IT

<u>from someone else</u> who has it, either directly or indirectly. Once you have been infected, recurrences are likely.

SYMPTOMS

The affected area will be <u>red, itchy, and scaly</u>. The infection may progress in a widening circular pattern—hence the name ringworm—with a clearing center of new skin.

WHAT IT DOES

Tinea cruris—a subgroup of tinea corporis, or ringworm of the body—is a fungus that grows only in dead, moist tissue. (Occasionally jock itch is caused by candida.) Redness and itching are caused by metabolic by-products of the fungus, which uses the skin as a culture medium. Antibody activity to this infection is not well understood.

Tinea will become asymptomatic and then be periodically reactivated when conditions are favorable for overgrowth. Complications arise from secondary infection from scratching.

DIAGNOSIS

- **by inspection**
- **by sampling** the infected skin (scraping) and looking at it under a microscope

TREATMENT

There are any number of <u>nonprescription products</u> on the market for the treatment of jock itch; in particularly stubborn cases, you will want to see a dermatologist, who can provide you with stronger medication.

Most important in the <u>prevention</u> of a reactivated infection is proper hygiene, and especially keeping the area dry and free of irritation. Make sure jock straps (or panties, for that matter) do not bind, and that clothing is loose and "breathes." Cotton pajamas help absorb perspiration at night.

You will want to be certain that your pubic itching is not caused by crabs or scabies, so inspect yourself carefully for symptoms of these other infections.

THE ALL-CLEAR SIGNAL

when the inflammation is cleared and the itching stops. Many people use the mild fungicides that are available for jock itch routinely—especially in powder form—to discourage recurrences.

SPECIAL CONSIDERATIONS FOR MEN

You *can* give jock itch to a female sex partner, so refrain from coitus if you have an active case.

SPECIAL CONSIDERATIONS FOR WOMEN

Tinea *can* be contracted *on the vulva*, where there will be minimal scaling, but the same redness and itching. Tinea does not infect the vagina.

INFESTATIONS

Crabs

pubic lice (*Phthirus pubis,* or *Pediculus pubis*) that are particular to human beings and most likely to be found in the groin area

THINGS YOU NEED TO KNOW

- Crabs can't really hurt you, but they are pretty repulsive. They are—unfortunately—easy to get, and—fortunately—easy to get rid of.
- It is hard to mistake a case of crabs for anything else, even if you've messed yourself up with too much scratching: you can *see* the little suckers, and they look like . . . crabs.
- People have different amounts of itchiness in response to an infestation by crabs, from much to almost none. Itchiness is usually as much a result of an allergic reaction to their bites as to their actually strolling around and generally making themselves at home.
- If you have crabs, you must be very certain to wash (with hot water) or dry clean all clothes and bedding.

WHERE YOU CATCH THEM

Pubic lice like pubic hair best, but they may also take up residence in other body hair, particularly in the underarms. If chil-

123

dren get them from an infected parent, they will be found on eyelashes and eyebrows and at the hairline. Occasionally an adult will also have eye infestation. They do not get into head hair.

HOW YOU CATCH THEM

from coming in contact with some place they are living, or some place they are passing through: another person, bed sheets or sleeping bag, clothing, perhaps even that maligned toilet seat. Crabs can only survive a couple of days out of contact with their source of nourishment . . . which is people.

SYMPTOMS

may begin shortly after contact (if you are particularly sensitive to the bites) but you usually do not begin to itch for about a **week to 10 days.** (Some people do not itch at all, although they may have many crabs.) The itching comes from the lice crawling around, as well as an allergic reaction to their bites.

A later symptom may be bluish spots—especially on the thighs —caused by tiny scabs and fecal deposits under the skin.

Tiny bloody spots in your underpants are also a sign of crabs.

WHAT THEY DO

Crabs are usually seen at the base of hairs, which is a convenient place to attach themselves between meals of your blood. They also lay their eggs there, cementing them with a substance called chitin.

A pubic louse lives for about a month, but its reproductive cycle is about 2 weeks: Eggs hatch in 8 days, and it takes an additional 8 days for the baby louse to begin to lay its own eggs.

The major complication of crab infestation—aside from potential allergic reactions—is secondary infection from scratching.

DIAGNOSIS

Crabs can be seen . . . if you are looking for them. They are grayish-brown (although they may have a reddish tinge if they have just finished a meal), and are about the size of a pinhead. If you catch them moving, you will see their legs. Otherwise they look like tiny skin moles.

The egg cases (nits) of the pubic louse are also easy to see where they are fastened at the base of hairs. They look like minute shiny seeds, and you will find them very hard to pull off, although they may be slid up the hair and removed that way.

Sometimes you have to be patient and look *very* carefully for the adults if you suspect you have crabs. The egg cases can sometimes be seen more easily, as they don't have legs and can't run and hide. The nits can also be felt if you run a fingernail up a hair from the base.

TREATMENT

There are two ways of dealing with crabs: directly and with a chemical wash.

Because crabs are something that most people do not want to wait one moment to be rid of, you will probably want to pick off as many as you can (you can use tweezers or fingers) as soon as you figure out that you have them. A pretty thorough job can be done this way, with both the crabs and their nits. Don't shave; but you may want to clip the pubic hairs somewhat to make the search-and-destroy mission a little easier.

You will want to finish the job by getting a prescription from your doctor for Kwell, which comes in both lotion and shampoo form—although the shampoo is most frequently used for crabs. (Over-the-counter products do not contain the active ingredient in Kwell, which is only available by prescription, and while the over-the-counters can be used in a pinch, Kwell is what works best.)

Directions for use of the shampoo are included with it; usually one wash is sufficient, but your doctor may recommend a second wash or an application of Kwell lotion. (This kills both the adults and the nits. Remaining nits—which should be translucent white because the baby crab is dead—must also be pulled off. Combing with a fine-toothed comb will get out dead adults.) You may want to wash once more in a week, to reassure yourself that any nits that may have escaped and hatched are dead.

Kwell has toxic ingredients, so do not use it more than suggested: there is such a thing as overkill.

Wash any clothes or sheets you have come into contact with in hot water, or send them to the dry cleaner.

THE ALL-CLEAR SIGNAL

Itching (from sensitization) may continue for a week or so *after* the crabs themselves are gone. If you have used the Kwell, and inspected yourself carefully and found nothing, consider yourself cured.

SPECIAL CONSIDERATIONS FOR PREGNANT WOMEN

As with any drug with toxic side effects, pregnant women should be especially careful with Kwell. Ask your doctor if it is all right to use it.

Scabies

a skin infection caused by the parasitic mite *Sarcoptes scabiei*

THINGS YOU NEED TO KNOW

- Scabies, unlike crabs, is not easily visible. You must deduce that you have it by the skin eruptions and itching that are the result of infestation.
- Scabies is highly contagious, and it is acquired by intimate contact—although this contact does not have to be explicitly sexual. In other words, if one person in the family is infected, everybody probably is and everybody must be treated.
- As is true with crabs, most of the discomfort and itching of scabies comes from allergic sensitization to the infestation, rather than from the mite itself.
- Scabies can look like a number of other skin conditions—including other allergic reactions and secondary syphilis—so it is important to be sure of the diagnosis.

WHERE YOU CATCH IT

anywhere below the neck (it is very unusual for scabies to ascend to the face and scalp). The pattern of infestation depends to some extent on how advanced the infection is when you first notice it: it usually starts in the groin area and spreads from there.

HOW YOU CATCH IT

through intimate—and often sexual—contact. Scabies can also be transmitted via infested clothing or bedding. For this reason you must wash everything an infected person has come into contact with, or send it to the dry cleaners.

SYMPTOMS

are likely to appear about **3 weeks** after exposure. *Reinfections* can have immediate symptoms (because of prior allergic sensitization). Symptoms are:

- itching, especially at night
- burrows—red or grayish-white ridges caused by the female mite tunneling through the skin to lay her eggs, and found where the skin is thin and/or delicate, such as the insides of the elbows, the wrists, and the webs of the fingers. Burrows may be present—but are less noticeable—around the waist, genitals, buttocks, and breasts.
- red bumps and/or sores—caused by the male mite. These are most frequently noticed on the trunk and arms.

WHAT IT DOES

The mite that causes scabies burrows into the skin and lives on blood. The female lays her eggs in tunnels she makes through the skin: they hatch in about 4 days. The larvae break out of the burrow, travel across the skin, and enter hair follicles, where—after they reach sexual maturity (about 18 days)—the cycle starts over again.

The major complication of scabies is secondary skin infection from scratching. Someone who has scabies for a period of time without knowing it is likely to have a *dermatitis*—a scaly, itchy, possibly oozing skin infection.

DIAGNOSIS

If you have never had scabies before, and are not sure of what to look for, be sure to see a doctor who *does* (more frequently a dermatologist then a gynecologist or urologist) and who will be able to recognize the syndrome.

A burrow can be scraped to retrieve a mite for microscopic inspection to confirm the diagnosis.

It is important to be sure that scabies *is* what you have, as there are other infections that have similar symptoms.

TREATMENT

Your doctor will give you detailed instructions, but the usual treatment for scabies involves bathing carefully and the use of Kwell lotion and/or shampoo.

If the sores or bumps have become infected, other medication may be necessary.

Don't neglect to treat any intimates (sexual and familial) and to wash out (with hot water) or dry-clean bedding, clothing, and surfaces that you have been in contact with.

THE ALL-CLEAR SIGNAL

Following prescribed treatment with lotion or shampoo should completely clear up the infestation.

However, because of allergic sensitization, you *may* itch for a number of weeks after treatment is complete. If you have followed treatment instructions and have carefully seen to it that people to whom you are close, as well as your enviornment, have been taken care of, you should not have to worry about reinfections.

SPECIAL CONSIDERATIONS FOR PREGNANT WOMEN

Kwell has toxic side effects, and should not be used without explicit permission from your obstetrician.

PROTOZOAN INFECTIONS

trichomoniasis • (intestinal protozoa are discussed under
INTESTINAL INFECTIONS)

PROTOZOA

are animals rather than plants: they move and eat, unlike plants, which stay still and make their own food. While protozoa are microscopic (or near-microscopic) single-cell organisms, they exhibit all the metabolic functions of higher animals. Some protozoa are parasitic (which means that they cannot live without the host, whom they may harm, and certainly do not help) to human beings.

Flagellates are a subgroup of protozoa (amoebas, for instance, are part of another subgroup); they have oval bodies and long whiplike tails that help them swim.

A trichomonad is one kind of flagellate.

Trichomoniasis

an infection caused by the protozoan parasite *Trichomonas vaginalis*

THINGS YOU NEED TO KNOW

- Trich (as it is frequently called) is a very common sexual infection among women, and responsible for a large proportion of vaginitis cases. At any given time, probably three million women have trich. In some groups, infection rates are as high as 40%.
- Trichomonads (the name of the organism) often coexist with other vaginal infections, so trich should always be considered in cases of vaginitis. Trich can also mask other infections: the majority of women who have gonorrhea, for instance, also have trich.
- While trich is basically a vaginal infection, men can be carriers, with silent cases. Trich *may* cause urethritis in men, and about 10% of men will have a penile discharge. Using condoms is usually adequate protection against a trich infection.
- Because of this "silence" in men, the recurrence of trichomoniasis in a woman is almost always owing to reinfection by a sexual partner. Therefore, if you are diagnosed as having trich, **your partner should *always* be treated.**
- The trichomonad can survive on a warm wet surface for some hours. Therefore, *while it is unlikely,* trich *can* legitimately be contracted from a bench in a locker room, shared clothing or douching equipment, or the famous toilet seat.

WHERE YOU CATCH IT

mucus-producing membranes
Women   vagina (vaginitis)
           cervix (cervicitis)
           urethra and bladder (cystitis)
Men   urethra (urethritis)
           prostate (prostatitis)
           seminal vesicles

HOW YOU CATCH IT

- sexual contact
- a warm wet surface that has infected secretions on it

FIRST SYMPTOMS

can appear **up to 4 weeks** after contact, but many infections are asymptomatic, especially in men.

Women
- vaginal discharge that may be
  heavy
  itchy
  foamy
  irritating
  yellowish, grayish, or greenish
  bad-smelling
- vagina and vulva look wet and inflamed
- rash on the cervix ("strawberry cervix")
- pain during coitus/lower abdominal pain
- the tendency to get worse right after menstruation

Men **(when there are symptoms)**
- itching
- thin, whitish discharge
- pain on urination
- smelly, irritating material under the foreskin

WHAT IT DOES

The trichomonad is a parasite that lives off substances present in the area of invasion. The organisms, in large numbers, have a toxic effect on tissue, and can cause extensive damage, eroding the mucosal surface and making it tender and inflamed.

Trichomonads cannot survive at a normal vaginal pH, which is slightly acid (see discussion of vaginal pH in the For Women Section in Part III), so to a great extent it is the ecology of the vagina that determines the pathogenicity of the infection. Optimal pH for a colonization by trichomonads is from 5.5 to 6.0. Healthy vaginal pH is below 5.0. (This is also why the post-menstrual period is especially susceptible to trich invasion.)

DIAGNOSIS

- **Culture** is the most reliable method. *Results:* 5 days.
- **Wet-mount smears** are quick, inexpensive, and reliable for positive identification (meaning that you can *confirm* a diagnosis of trich, but cannot rule one out). Specimens are taken from the vagina of the woman, and from the urethra of the man. Prostatic secretions (one component of semen) can also be examined. The parasites may be clearly visible under a microscope, swimming around propelled by their little flagellae. *Results:* immediate.

TREATMENT

Killing these little animals requires more drastic measures than killing other microbes, and there is only one sure cure: Flagyl (metronidazole), usually by mouth, but occasionally used topically. New research indicates that one big dose is as effective as the old 7-day regimen . . . and it has fewer side effects.

However, you want to be *absolutely certain* that you *have* trich before being treated for it: Flagyl's side effects can be unpleasant (nausea and vomiting, headache, an intolerance to alcohol), and it has been accused of having carcinogenic properties (although this has yet to be conclusively demonstrated; and such concerns must be secondary to cure if the infection does exist). This means that *unless the trichomonads have been identified in wet-mount, you will want to wait for the results of the culture to be treated.* **Don't take Flagyl until a trich infection has been *positively* identified.** Doctors may also prescribe something to restore the vaginal pH and help the damaged tissue heal.

Women who are susceptible to trich infections or suspect that there is one coming on can sometimes head off a full-blown infection by douching, either with Betadine or with vinegar and water (2 tablespoons of white vinegar to a quart of warm water). But **do not douche before seeing your doctor; it washes away the evidence.**

Your sex partner must also be treated or you are very likely to be reinfected. Many doctors prescribe enough Flagyl for two as a matter of course.

THE ALL-CLEAR SIGNAL

You can consider yourself free of infection a week after taking your medication.

SPECIAL CONSIDERATIONS FOR WOMEN

- Trich can lurk around for quite a while in a subclinical state, waiting for vaginal pH to change to cause a real infection. For this reason it is sometimes hard to know just when an infection was contracted.
- Douching can set you up for trich by changing vaginal ecology . . . another good reason to avoid routine douching.
- **Recurrent trich infections can cause changes in the cervix that resemble pre-cancerous tissue** (carcinoma *in situ*). These changes are the most frequent cause of abnormal Pap smears.
- The discharge from **trichomoniasis can**—and often does—**mask gonorrhea and/or chlamydia.**
- There appears to be a complicated relationship between trich and herpes that is not yet fully understood.
- Women can easily—and regularly—be checked for trichomonads in the course of the routine Pap smear.

SPECIAL CONSIDERATIONS FOR PREGNANT WOMEN

Pregnant women and nursing mothers should not be taking Flagyl.

INTESTINAL INFECTIONS

*bacterial: shigellosis, salmonellosis • enteritis • protozoan:
giardiasis, amebiasis • infestations: pinworms*

Intestinal Infections

can be caused by a variety of organisms

THINGS YOU NEED TO KNOW

- While <u>intestinal infections</u> are not narrowly defined as sexually transmitted—and indeed, are transmitted in any number of ways—they <u>can be caught in the course of sexual contact through combinations of oral-anal-genital exposure</u> ... particularly when personal hygiene is less than exemplary.
- <u>Many intestinal infections are asymptomatic.</u> This means you can become a carrier—without knowing it—or be infected by a carrier.
- <u>Symptoms of intestinal infections vary from none to devastating.</u>
- <u>Intestinal disorders are in general difficult to diagnose</u>—and to distinguish from one another—but if you have a gastrointestinal disruption that hangs on—or makes you feel ill—beyond what you would expect for a garden-variety stomach flu or a transient bad reaction to something you ate, consider the possibility that you have been infected with a parasite or a bacterium ... *particularly* if anal contact is part of

your sexual repertoire. And get checked out even if you are reluctant to talk about your sexual practices to a doctor.

- Private physicians are often neither equipped for nor educated to the subtleties of diagnosing intestinal infections. Don't accept an "I-don't-know-let's-wait-and-see"; ask to be referred to a parasitology or tropical disease department in a local hospital. Or go to a public health clinic where they have seen other cases like yours.
- Don't allow yourself to be treated until you are sure of what you have. Each of these infections has a very specific cure.
- Being sure of what you have almost always requires what is known as a "warm stool" sample. Don't be deterred by the indelicacy of the diagnostic method—the people who are used to working in the field aren't embarrassed, and you shouldn't be.
- It is important to be aware that certain sexual practices—most particularly oral-anal sex—significantly increase your chances of picking up an intestinal infection. While such activities are more commonly a feature of male homosexual relationships, whenever anal eroticism is included in sex play, the participants may be exposed to these infections. This is also a situation in which personal hygiene *does* make a difference.

WHERE YOU CATCH THESE INFECTIONS

Initially these parasites and bacteria infect the gastrointestinal tract, but—depending on the organism—they may spread to other parts of the body.

HOW YOU CATCH THEM

Transmission *always* involves the ingestion of the organism in one of its forms (which may include cysts and eggs) from contaminated fecal matter. Oral contact, therefore, with any body part that may have these organisms on it (including hands and genitals), or with food or eating utensils handled by someone who is infected, is the path of infection.

SYMPTOMS

Symptoms vary in intensity (with many infections being asymptomatic) but they almost always include

- diarrhea

Other symptoms may be

- gas
- foul-smelling stools
- alternating diarrhea and constipation
- bloody, mucusy, watery, or greasy stools
- a bloated feeling
- stomach cramps

Intestinal infections can really . . . uh . . . take it out of you: anytime diarrhea is involved (which often means dehydration as well as a loss of electrolytes and minerals) you are going to feel as if you've been run over by a truck.

CATEGORIES OF INTESTINAL INFECTIONS

bacterial including—and most commonly—
shigellosis (caused by shigellae)
salmonellosis (caused by salmonellae, which are responsible for some types of dysentery)
enteritis (caused by *Campylobacter*)
In addition to intestinal symptoms, bacterial infections anywhere in the body are likely to cause fever and chills.

protozoan including
giardiasis (caused by *Giardia lamblia*)
amebiasis (caused by *Entamoeba histolytica*)
Transmitted as cysts, these parasites grow into adults and can be very debilitating.

infestations
usually pinworms, although other worm infections can be transmitted sexually.
Pinworms are highly contagious, and while you are likely to become infected by exposure to a child who has them (they are caught primarily through the "dirty hand" syndrome: playing somewhere—like a sandbox that may have contaminated animal feces in it—and then ingesting the eggs), pinworms can lay low a related group of people in short order. The rule is usually that if one person in the family has them, so will every-

one else. They can be picked up from clothing, bedding, hands, food, etc. They can even be inhaled.

Pinworms can also be transmitted sexually; they lay their eggs around the anus at night, and oral-genital contact with an infected person carries some risk of infection.

Pinworm symptoms can be serious in small children (who may even become convulsive), but in adults they are responsible only for intense itching around and just inside the anus—particularly at night, when the worms come out to lay their eggs. A child infected with pinworms can be checked by a parent with a flashlight at night: you can see the worms—which look like little white threads—in and around the anus. (Diagnosis can also be made by the "Scotch Tape test": tape is pressed against the unbathed anus in the morning and examined on a glass slide under a microscope for any pinworm eggs that may have been picked up.)

DIAGNOSIS

requires "warm stool" that can be inspected microscopically for parasites, or can be cultured for bacterial infection.

Don't take medicines or enemas before seeing the doctor: it makes it just that much harder to make an accurate diagnosis.

TREATMENT

Different drugs are used, of course, to treat different infections; antibiotics and Flagyl (metronidazole) are the two big guns. Be certain of diagnosis before you submit to treatment: neither class of drugs should be used carelessly.

Sometimes the treatment itself can make you feel unwell (especially Flagyl; see discussion in section on trichomoniasis), but it is important to follow your doctor's instructions exactly to make sure that the infection is completely eradicated. It is the nature of enteric infections that they can become harder to treat in subsequent cases.

Any sex partner(s) should be examined also. Because of the highly infectious nature of intestinal infections, they usually need to be treated.

THE ALL-CLEAR SIGNAL

It is not always easy to tell when an intestinal infection has been successfully treated. Repeat stool studies are necessary to be sure.

GENITAL INFECTIONS BY INTESTINAL BACTERIA

Intestinal bacteria which inoculate the vagina or urethra can cause infections (vaginitis, urethritis). These bacteria (*Escherichia coli* and other coliform bacteria) are very much at home in the intestinal tract but real troublemakers when they invade the delicate, vulnerable tissues of places where they do not naturally belong.

Women can protect themselves against such infections by being sure to wipe front to back after a bowel movement, by keeping clean, and by making sure that a male partner washes his penis carefully after anal intercourse and before attempting vaginal penetration.

Men can help protect themselves by urinating following anal penetration.

SPECIAL CONSIDERATIONS FOR HOMOSEXUAL MEN

Because of the kinds of sexual activity that homosexuals engage in, they are at relatively high risk for sexually transmitted intestinal infections (as well as for urethritis caused by enteric organisms). The incidence of such infections could be cut down if

- all basic hygienic measures were observed, and
- partners of infected men were informed and treated.

PART III

Your Sexual Health

FOR WOMEN

The Healthy Vagina

Mr. Rogers (of the children's show) sings a song to kids that goes, in part: "Boys are fancy on the outside; girls are fancy on the inside . . ." There is no question that basic anatomical differences make a boy much earlier and better acquainted with his own—and other boys'—genitals than a girl with hers, but a girl also has to contend with social conditioning that makes her uneasy at—and even repelled by—the thought of looking at or touching her sexual parts. Women still have trouble relating to what's "down there," and it is the rare woman who could draw and label a diagram of her reproductive organs, or even a drawing of her vulva. Examining your own vulva and vagina should be as simple and straightforward—and unself-conscious—an exercise as looking in your own (wet, dark) mouth . . . and it should be a primary health responsibility. Trouble almost always comes with its peculiar and particular signs, but even if you don't have an itch or a discharge or lower abdominal pain, you can get to know your body and its normal changes with a little practiced observation. Gynecological health is *your* responsibility, not just your doctor's.

Women who regard their genitals as an important, fascinating, and *accessible* part of themselves—and their sexuality as an ally of positive self-image rather than an enemy to outwit and gain control over—are more aware, more integrated, and healthier, in every way.

THINGS YOU SHOULD KNOW

- A healthy vagina doesn't itch, burn, or otherwise cause pain. It looks healthy. It smells healthy.
- A healthy vagina is a self-cleaning organ, like the eye. Like the eye it is naturally lubricated, which helps in the cleaning process, and, just as the eye tears occasionally, the vagina produces a normal *small* amount of discharge, which should be whitish and not have a foul odor. This normal discharge is made up of dead cells from the vaginal walls, products of the ovulatory cycle, cervical mucus, and vaginal transudate (the natural wetness that is necessary to protect the mucous membrane . . . and incidentally the same substance that as "lubrication" becomes more copious during sexual excitement).
- The vagina always has what is known as its natural "flora" (also called microflora) or "ecology"—a balance of bacterial and fungal organisms (balance is the operative concept) that keeps it healthy—much as is true of the mouth. Therefore, while cleanliness is of course a major issue in maintaining health, "ecological balance" in the vagina is even more important: once that balance is upset, it can be difficult to get it right again.
- Vaginal pH (the acid-alkali balance) also plays an essential role in maintaining a healthy vaginal ecology. The healthy vagina is slightly acid, with pH values from 4.0 to 5.0. You are much more susceptible to infection when the pH values of the vagina rise above 5.0—as they often do just before and just after menstruation, when the pH can rise to 6.0 or more. Infection in turn can cause a rise in the pH.
- A healthy vagina does not need a regular cleaning any more than the eye does. Furthermore, douching can and often does create more problems than it corrects: it upsets the delicate ecology of the vagina; it may force infection through the os (opening) of the cervix into the uterus, from where it can spread deeper into the pelvis; and allergic reac-

tions to douching solutions are not uncommon. Douching can also mask infections by washing away symptoms that would otherwise alert you to trouble.

If you *do* douche (and this should be infrequently, perhaps after your period or after having left a diaphragm in for too long), you do not need commercial preparations—unless they have specifically been prescribed by your doctor. The best general-purpose douche is 2 tablespoons of white vinegar in a quart of warm water. (Vinegar helps maintain the acid balance.) Just remember: every time you douche you wash away the good bacteria with the bad bacteria, leaving yourself open to infection (such as candidiasis, for example).

KEEPING TABS ON YOURSELF

There are three ways to monitor your own genital health (and thus your *general* health): how you feel, how you look, and how you smell. (Don't laugh. Smell is sometimes the most reliable of the senses when something is going on in your vagina.) The amount and color—as well as the smell—of any discharge are also good early indications of trouble.

If you suspect trouble, don't "wait and see." And *don't* self-treat . . . unless you are *very* sure of the nature of your problem, *and* have checked with your doctor.

HOW YOU FEEL

A general feeling of illness that cannot be traced to another source—especially if accompanied by fever and abdominal pain —can be a sign of sexual infection that has advanced to the "complication" stage. If such sensations co-occur with a discharge and a change in your vaginal odor, you can be pretty sure that you are dealing with a sexual infection. **See a doctor immediately.**

Discharge, itching, a heavy or uncomfortable feeling in the pelvis, and pain during coitus or urination are also signs of trouble. **Sexual infections almost never go away by themselves. If you have something, there is very little chance that you will get**

rid of it without treatment. It will not get better. And it can make you sick, sterile, or worse. This is no time for an attack of modesty, or to worry about being judged.

HOW YOU LOOK

You should know what your **vulva and perineum** (and anus) look like, and you should get used to inspecting *at least* your external genitalia regularly with a mirror and a good strong light. If there is anything that feels or looks funny, or that hurts or itches, or more than usual vaginal discharge, you should see your doctor. Your own inspection of yourself can be the first line of defense against warts, chancres, HSV-2 blisters, and other kinds of sores.

You should know what your **vagina and cervix** look like, just as you should know what your tongue and teeth and gums look like. Many women cannot imagine actually looking inside themselves and seeing their own vaginas and cervices, and this is understandable, considering the artificial and exaggerated delicacy and helplessness with which most of us view our bodies. However, there are more and more good reasons for a woman to try to get over her distaste and fear and to learn to take responsibility—at least in part—for her own health. The women's self-help movement has encouraged such knowledge, and has paved the way for more mainstream acceptance of a woman's fundamental *right*—as well as *responsibility*—to know more about her own body and its functioning and to be an active partner in any diagnosis and treatment.

Until the women's health movement insisted on this more direct involvement in one's own health, a woman found it downright impossible to get a look inside herself, unless she had a friendly, liberal doctor who positioned her right and gave her a mirror so that she could observe her own pelvic exam. Now there are disposable plastic specula (rather than those unfriendly and complicated-looking steel instruments the doctor uses: a speculum is the instrument the gynecologist uses to hold apart the walls of the vagina so that the cervix can be seen) available to anyone who is willing to track them down; they can sometimes be found at surgical supply houses, sometimes in drugstores, but

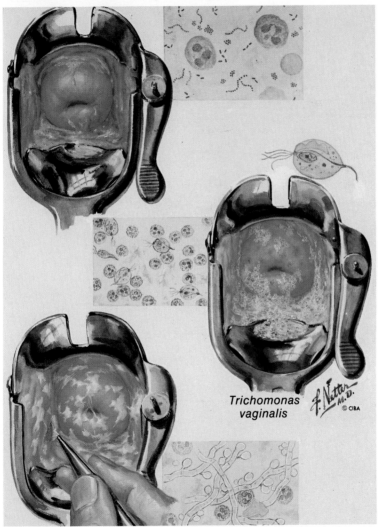

Hemophilus vaginalis (Gardnerella vaginalis),
one cause of so-called nonspecific vaginitis

Trichomonas vaginalis

Candida albicans (yeast infection)

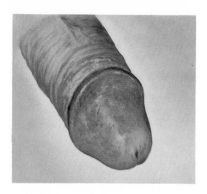

Balanitis: inflammation of
the head of the penis,
usually by *Candida*

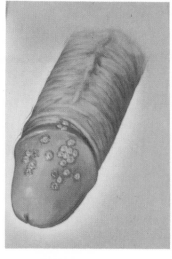

HSV-2 blisters

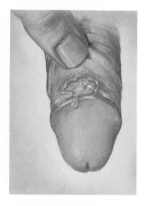

Chancroid chancre

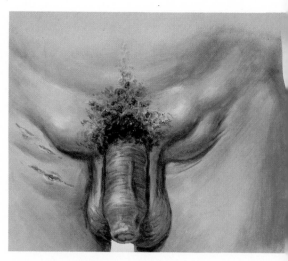

Lymphogranuloma venereum, caused by one
strain of *Chlamydia (C. trachomatis)*

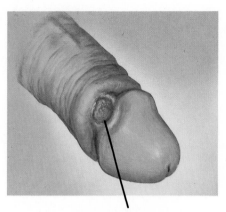

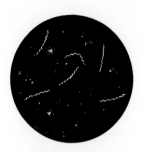

Syphilis spirochetes

Syphilis chancres

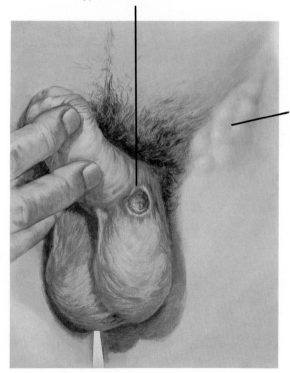

Swollen
lymph nodes

© CIBA

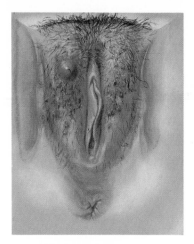

Sebaceous cysts,
occluded hair follicles

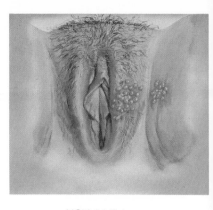

HSV-2 blisters

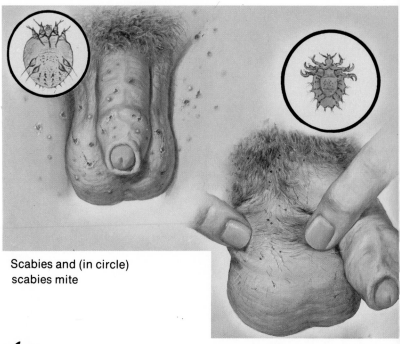

Scabies and (in circle)
scabies mite

Crabs (infestation by pubic lice)

© CIBA

you can always find out where to get them through a local women's center or your doctor.

Why is it important to be able to see your cervix? Because not only do significant changes take place on a monthly basis, but certain sexual infections are more likely to manifest themselves on—or through—the cervix than anywhere else; gonorrhea and trichomoniasis are only two examples. Sexual infections often have telltale signs—pus, lesions, inflammation—that are readily visible if you just look.

Besides . . . it's damn interesting.

Use of a Speculum

A speculum has two rounded bladelike extensions fixed together on a hinge. The speculum is inserted into the vagina in its closed position, and then opened by pressing the handle and lever on its protruding parts together (it's easy to figure out when you see the speculum) so that the vaginal walls are held apart and you can get a good view of the cervix. You will also need a strong light source and a decent-sized mirror, as well as some practice with the correct angling of both so that you can see easily. So take the time and practice: It is something you should be doing regularly for the rest of your life. *It could be argued that knowing how to use a speculum, and knowing what to look for when it is in use, is as important for a woman as knowing how to examine her own breasts.*

There are a number of books that discuss vaginal health—as well as other aspects of women's particular sexual health problems—and that explain in detail how to use a speculum and what to look for. A good up-to-date one is *A New View of a Woman's Body,* by the Federation of Feminist Women's Health Centers (Simon and Schuster, 1981), which has especially good illustrations. You might also ask your doctor to give you a lesson in the use of a speculum, and ask him/her what s/he suggests you look for, and how often to examine yourself. Briefly, however, speculum use goes like this:

Situate yourself so that you can conveniently juggle your speculum, your light source, and a mirror (a little standing mirror makes this easier, as does a high-intensity lamp with an adjustable arm that you shine into the *mirror* so that it throws light into the vagina). You will be acquainted with the speculum already

145

from visits to the gynecologist, but you can experiment with yours to familiarize yourself with its open and closed positions. The speculum can be inserted in any direction (some sources suggest putting it in sideways—as that may be more comfortable —and then turning it), but the blades should end up in an up/down position—that is, against the forward (toward the bladder) and back (toward the rectum) walls of the vagina. (Make sure you get the speculum all the way in before opening it up; it should go as deep as the hinge.) It is important to be relaxed when you open the speculum or you will have quite a job—remember how strong the vaginal muscles are! A doctor will insert the speculum with its crooked handle down; you may want to put the crooked handle up, as it's easier to look inside yourself when it is in this position. Try both and do what works best for you.

When the speculum is properly inserted—and open, of course —you should be able to see the cervix pretty easily. It is a good idea to get used to examining yourself as often as once a week in the beginning. This way you can become familiar with normal cyclical changes and you will notice immediately if something seems to be awry.

HOW YOU SMELL

Smell is the great lost sense in our overdeodorized, powdered, and perfumed modern world; but smell is the oldest and the most acute sense, and—at least in some species—the sense most crucial to the maintenance of normal mating behavior. (For instance, if you destroy a rat's capacity to smell, it can no longer function sexually.)

One of the best ways to keep tabs on your health is to be familiar with your own vaginal odor, and to be *immediately* suspicious if that odor changes and/or gets foul. (A healthy vagina *smells* healthy and clean without the benefit of deodorization, just as a healthy mouth should smell healthy and clean without mouthwash.) Some cases of vaginitis have specific smells (see vaginitis chart) that may be diagnostic and at the very least indicate that something is wrong. Also, smell is sometimes the only way that an otherwise asymptomatic infection betrays itself.

This is a good place to mention a couple of common reasons for foul-smelling discharge that have nothing to do with infection: (1) the wearing of nonabsorbent fabrics that hold the *normal* discharge against the body so that it putrefies (another sound reason for making sure that whatever you wear has a cotton crotch); and (2) a bad memory for tampons and diaphragms left in place, which also trap normal secretions that subsequently (and odorifically) decay.

And while you are checking out normal healthy vaginal smell, check out your normal discharge. Recognize how the consistency and "feel" of the secretions change during your menstrual cycle as the cervical mucus changes, and how it is more or less cloudy. (Cervical mucus examination is also increasingly used in the rhythm birth-control method.) Normal discharge can be observed on the cervix as well.

So keep tabs on yourself. Cures are all fine, but the best way to take care of yourself is to *prevent* problems by a heightened awareness of what it is to be healthy. Some of these techniques may make you uncomfortable (psychologically, not physically), but a sexual infection is going to make you even more uncomfortable (psychologically *and* physically).

Vaginitis

If you have a vagina, at some time in your life—and very likely *more* than once—it will be inflamed as the result of some infection, change of vaginal ecology, or allergic reaction. Usually a vaginitis is easily put right and there is nothing to worry about, but occasionally vaginitis can be an indication of more serious problems.

THE BIG THREE

While the great majority of the infections covered in this book can at some point cause a vaginitis, the most commonly seen vaginitises are **Hemophilus vaginalis** (or HV), a bacterial infection; **trichomoniasis** (or trich), a protozoan infection; and **candidiasis** (sometimes called moniliasis), a fungus infection: the "itch triumvirate."

You should be aware that the *presence* of one or more of these organisms is not necessarily the same thing as an *infection* by the organism; in fact, all the above as well as some others (and *always Candida*) may be present in small numbers in the healthy vagina, where they are kept in check by the body's resistance to infection.

In many women, any given incident of vaginitis may be caused by more than one organism *(multi-agent).* Studies demonstrate widely varying figures, but it would be fair to say that half of any group of women (and sometimes more than 80%) will be harboring at least *one* organism in concentrations great enough to cause infection under certain circumstances—psychological and physical stresses, including trauma associated with overenthusiastic coitus (sometimes called friction-rub syndrome), antibiotic therapy, illness, and fatigue.

Organisms can also mask each other, so there may be a silent case of PID-causing chlamydia or gonorrhea lurking under cover of a vaginitis with more obvious symptoms.

THE INFAMOUS "NONSPECIFIC" (NSV)

Nonspecific vaginal infections (usually, but not always, bacterial) used to be the great catch-all category, into which everything that didn't immediately identify itself (or that the doctor was too lazy to go after) was dumped. Nonspecifics were treated with a broad-spectrum antibiotic in the hope that they would clear up, and sometimes they did. Then again, sometimes they didn't.

We now know that it is not enough to get this blitz treatment and hope that it is going to work, because the truth of the matter is that no infection is *really* nonspecific: infections are caused by identifiable organisms that have names . . . and what's more important, that have quite specific treatments (**HV** and **chlamydia** are two biggies that have recently been cut out of this "no-name" pack). This means that if you are told you have NSV, you should ask some incisive questions, and make sure that everything possible has been done to identify and treat a *specific* organism. Very few infections can be accurately diagnosed just by sight— or *completely* diagnosed, since so many infections mask other infections—and need other diagnostic techniques to confirm clinical impressions.

Diagnostic steps should include:

- *minimal* confirmation by **wet-mount smear** in the doctor's office. (This involves taking a small sample of the vaginal secretions, putting it on a glass slide, and looking at it right there, in the doctor's office.) There are other kinds of smears that are sent to a lab, but a wet-mount must be looked at under a microscope as soon as it is taken. (The Big Three are often readily apparent in a wet-mount.)
- *further* confirmation can—and often should—be made by **laboratory culture,** especially in a difficult-to-cure case. (A sample of vaginal secretions is wiped onto a growth medium and then sent to a lab.) For reasons that should be self-evident by now (having to do with masking of more serious infections, and inadequate and/or mistaken treatment that can further mask), **you should never accept a "blitz" treatment until it has been established that your vaginitis is either caused by multiple organisms (multi-agent) or that it is caused by an organism for which a "broad-spectrum" antibiotic is suitable treatment.** *Occasionally* a doctor will appropriately diagnose by deduction, as must frequently be done with chlamydia, for which there is no cheap, easily available diagnostic test. Just be certain that any therapy is explained, and that you understand *why* you are being treated with the drug(s) your doctor chooses.

Some Other Specific "Nonspecifics"

The vagina can be colonized by any number of different bacteria that do not belong in it and consequently can cause infection. Basically it is a case of wandering germs that can be responsible not only for vaginitis but for a whole range of other "-itises" (see General Categories of Female Infections), some of them chronic. Sexual activity, or another infection already present, makes it more likely that organisms in the wrong place will become a full-blown infection. The most common bacteria with which this can happen are *E. coli (Escherichia coli)* or other coliform bacteria. These are from the gut, or intestinal tract, and are spread to the vagina either as a result of auto-contamination—wiping in the wrong direction, for instance—or from anal penetration and then vaginal penetration without washing the penis or fingers between the two.

<u>Streptococcus</u> and <u>staphylococcus</u> infections also can be spread to the vagina from fingers, other skin surfaces, or sometimes oral-genital contact.

A last word of caution: not only do these "nonspecifics" *mimic* other infections, but they may *mask* them. In short, <u>the culprit organism should be tracked down before treatment.</u>

ALLERGIES

No discussion of vaginitis is complete without mentioning allergies; too often what is erroneously treated as an infection is really an allergic reaction (a local immune response) that is usually characterized by itching and/or hives and redness, but may also involve more serious inflammation. Among the frequent culprits are: douche solutions, deodorized tampons, jellies and foams, bubble bath, talcum powder (use cornstarch instead), fingernail polish, and perfume or cologne. Less frequently a woman may have an allergic reaction to certain bacteria, or possibly even be selectively sensitized to certain men's semen.

Allergic reactions frequently distinguish themselves from a true infection by appearing shortly after exposure to the allergen; disease does not come on quite so quickly.

A good rule to follow is not to use any substance on, in, or around the vaginal area that is not necessary to your health or to the business of contraception.

General Categories of Female Infections

VAGINITIS

is inflammation of the vagina, often accompanied by discharge and itching, and can be caused by:

- *Hemophilus vaginalis* (HV)
- chlamydia
- trichomoniasis
- candidiasis

- *E. coli* and other coliform bacteria
- strep or staph infections
- allergies

As a *general* rule, HV is the smelliest, trich has the most discharge, and candida itches most. These infections may mask either gonorrhea or chlamydia. (See vaginitis/cervicitis chart.)

CERVICITIS

is inflammation of the cervix, usually caused by:
- gonorrhea
- chlamydia
- trichomoniasis
- HSV-2 (herpes simplex virus type II, or genital herpes)

A vaginitis may obscure a cervicitis, although anything that infects the vagina may also potentially infect the cervix. Cervicitis can either be local or an indication of an infection deeper in the reproductive organs . . . in the tubes, for instance. (See vaginitis/cervicitis chart.)

SALPINGITIS

is infection of the tube through which eggs pass from the ovary to the uterus, usually caused by PID (pelvic inflammatory disease) that is in turn caused by either chlamydia or gonorrhea. These and associated secondary infections may leave scars which prevent the movement of the egg and may cause sterility or ectopic pregnancy (development of the embryo in the fallopian tube rather than the uterus, which can lead to rupture of the tube and fatal hemorrhage).

PID (PELVIC INFLAMMATORY DISEASE)

is a serious health problem for women that is misdiagnosed in more than a third of all cases, and is responsible for infertility, ectopic pregnancy, endometritis, ovarian cysts, and abscesses. It is almost always caused by either chlamydial or gonorrheal infection, both of which are frequently asymptomatic in women; indeed, the first indication of infection by either of these organisms may be the PID itself. (Pelvic abscesses sometimes seen

VAGINITIS/CERVICITIS

	DISCHARGE (IF PRESENT)	FOUL SMELL	VULVAL ITCH	VAGINAL INFLAM- MATION OR RASH
HV	heavy white	fishy	little	rashy
candi- diasis	white cheesy		usually severe	✔
trichomoniasis	yellowish frothy copious	✔	mild to severe	✔
chlamydia	pus-like or watery			
gonorrhea	pus-like thick yellow			
cervical HSV-2	✔		only with vulval lesions	

following surgery or in women wearing IUDs are frequently caused by other organisms, like *E. coli* and bacteroides.)

PID frequently becomes a chronic problem. **There will be almost one million cases of pelvic infection this year, and 100,000 women**—most quite young—**will be permanently sterilized** by PID in the same period of time.

Symptoms of PID include:

- fever
- *bilateral* lower abdominal pain
- vaginal discharge (may be pus-like or bloody)
- pelvic tenderness and painful coitus
- high white cell count in the blood
- nausea and vomiting

The IUD is associated with an approximately four times greater risk of PID, especially for women under 30. (See discussion of the IUD in the later section on contraception.)

URETHRITIS/ PAINFUL URINATION	CERVICITIS	PAINFUL COITUS	LOWER ABDOM- INAL PAIN	SPREADS TO TUBES (STERILITY)
		✔		
		✔		
✔	"straw- berry cervix"	✔	✔	
✔ (occasion- ally)	✔	✔	✔	✔
✔ (occasion- ally)	granular erosions	✔	✔	✔
only with vulval lesions	✔	✔	✔	

✔ = may be present

CYSTITIS AND URETHRITIS

are inflammations of the urethra and bladder. Because the female urethra is considerably shorter than that of the male, women are more vulnerable to bladder infections, which are caused by:

- *E. coli* and other coliform bacteria
- trichomoniasis
- chlamydia
- gonorrhea
- herpes (which causes a kind of "mock" cystitis, but may evolve into real cystitis in cases of urinary retention)

Bladder infections can make a woman very uncomfortable and can cause complications and ascend to the kidneys if left untreated. The symptoms of a bladder infection (which implies a prior urethral infection) are:

- a constant sensation of having to urinate
- painful urination
- general feeling of fatigue and illness, and possibly fever
- a "thudding" sensation when the bladder is emptied

Conditions which predispose a woman to cystitis include:

- wiping in the wrong direction, so that fecal matter gets into the urethra
- general lack of hygiene, or the lack of hygiene of a sex partner
- irritation of the urethral opening during coitus (sometimes called "honeymoon cystitis")
- urine retention, if the bladder does not drain well, or enough liquids are not drunk to flush the bladder and urethra continually
- the introduction of a large number of infectious organisms
- childbirth
- bladder catheterization

Other Things Women Worry About

We briefly mention the following infections/conditions because while they are *not* in any way sexually transmitted, they are sometimes confused with and/or potentiated by a sexual infection, and you should be familiar with each of them.

ENDOMETRIOSIS

is commonly misdiagnosed as PID (if antibiotic therapy does not clear up the symptoms, you may have endometriosis).

Endometriosis is a **leading cause of infertility in women over 25** and the second most common gynecological problem in the U.S. after fibroid tumors. As many as 8 million women may have it, and a pitifully small proportion of these are correctly diagnosed.

Because it is a condition in which tissue from the lining of the uterus is found growing in the abdominal cavity, symptoms of endometriosis become more severe during the menstrual period, with pain and bleeding. Between periods a woman may experience painful coitus and lower abdominal discomfort.

Endometriosis can be treated—sometimes by surgery. Any abdominal pain of some duration should be investigated, and endometriosis should always be considered.

TOXIC SHOCK SYNDROME (TSS)

is caused by a poisonous strain of an organism called *Staphylococcus aureus,* and is seen most frequently although not exclusively in young menstruating women who use tampons, particularly those of the "super-absorbent" type.

The exact mechanism of toxic shock in these cases is not yet understood, but it seems to have something to do with breakdown of materials in the tampons interacting with menstrual blood to create a culture medium for the bacteria which are present already in the vagina. These bacteria typically release toxins which may be responsible for many of TSS's symptoms.

Between 500 and 1,000 cases of TSS are reported every year, but it seems clear that five to ten times as many cases may go undiagnosed. For those women who have had one attack and have not been treated specifically for TSS, there is a high likelihood of a second, potentially more severe episode.

Symptoms of TSS include some or any of the following:

- sudden high fever
- rash
- vomiting
- diarrhea
- shock . . . and death

The best protection you can provide yourself is to avoid using tampons, especially those of the super-absorbent type. If you *must* use tampons, be certain to change them frequently.

Pregnant women should not use tampons at all.

CANCER

This is what we know about cancer and sexual activity:

- Women who have multiple sex partners have a higher rate of cervical cancer than women with none or few.

This is what we know about <u>cancer and sexual infections:</u>

- Women who have recurrent HSV-2 infections of the cervix have a cervical cancer rate five to ten times higher than women who do not.
- A quarter of women who have recurrent HSV-2 show—over time—cervical changes consistent with pre-malignant states.
- Recurrent trichomoniasis infections can cause changes in the cervix that resemble pre-cancerous tissue.
- Venereal warts on the cervix have certain pre-malignant characteristics.

However, no *causal* relationships have been established. Any woman who considers herself at high risk should have Pap smears more frequently—every six months—to monitor any change in cells of the cervix. Such cervical changes can be treated.

THINGS *NOT* TO WORRY ABOUT

- **sebaceous cysts/occluded hair follicles,** which can cause small hard bumps under the skin, or pimplelike eruptions. But your doctor should see and diagnose these.
- **leukorrhea,** a light, pasty-white, non-smelly discharge that is a product of the natural self-cleansing action of the vagina. Leukorrhea *can* begin to seem like something nasty if you wear nonabsorbent and/or tight underwear or pantyhose.
- **cyclical changes.** At mid-cycle (ovulation) a mucus-like vaginal secretion is normal and healthy.

What to Look for in a Male Partner

Women have the advantage when it comes to protecting themselves; symptoms of a sexual infection are usually much more obvious in a man than in a woman.

- Obvious <u>**sores, bumps, or lumps**</u> should be considered suspicious . . . and this is not the time to be polite. If you see—or feel—something that concerns you, *ask.* You may do *him* a favor by calling his attention to something he has not yet noticed. If he doesn't have an immediate—and plausible—explanation (like a wayward zipper) for some suspicious imperfection, **don't have sexual contact.** Some men do have small pearly bumps all around the edge of the head of the penis. These are *penile papules* and are neither infectious nor harmful.

- It is possible to check subtly for **discharge** during sex play. The small amount of lubrication provided by the Cowper's glands is much like a woman's—colorless, odorless, and slick—and this natural lubrication will appear in droplets at the urethral opening during sexual excitation. Any secretion that is smelly or opaque (obviously excluding the semen itself, which is ejaculated during orgasm, and rarely "leaks" before it) should be cause for you to reconsider sexual contact.

- Simple cleanliness is something that should be required of any sex partner—not only of his genitals (and he should clean especially carefully around and under his foreskin, if he has one) but of his hands. Many are the vaginal infections that have come from dirty hands during sex play. In other words, if you wouldn't put it in your mouth, don't put it in your vagina. (Your mouth is dirtier anyway.)

Contraception

This is not the place to go into a detailed discussion of contraceptive choices, but there are some things you should know about them as they relate to sexual infections.

ABOUT THE PILL

Effects of the Pill are mixed, but there is one thing that can be said for sure: since women (and their partners) have discarded barrier contraceptives in favor of nonbarrier methods, the frequency of sexual infections has increased greatly. That is the single most important thing to know about the Pill.

As for the Pill itself:

- While the rates of chlamydia and venereal warts are higher for those women taking oral contraceptives, the rates of gonorrhea, trichomoniasis, and candida appear to be the same.

- The Pill may predispose a woman to cervicitis because of increased exposure of cervical glands.
- *However,* the progesterone in the Pill may provide some protection against PID because of the mucus plug it supports in the cervical opening.

ABOUT THE IUD

There is evidence that the IUD (intrauterine device) increases susceptibility to infection, both because it sets up a mild irritation in the uterus making an existing infection worse, and because infection can climb up the string (which hangs into the vagina) into the uterus—a sort of highway for bacteria. This was especially true with the now out-of-favor Dalkon Shield, which had a multi-filament string. **Always have a complete workup for sexual infections (including gonorrhea, syphilis, and trichomoniasis) before having an IUD inserted.**

The IUD does not protect against tubal (ectopic) pregnancies, and because of the greater risk of PID in women who have IUDs (PID can cause tubal damage that impedes the progress of the fertilized egg), there is a consequent compounded risk of an ectopic pregnancy and its attendant dangers.

ABOUT BARRIER METHODS

These include the **condom, diaphragm,** and **cervical cap,** and the **foams, jellies, and creams** used either alone or in conjunction with them.

People who use barrier methods of contraception have lower rates of every single one of the sexual infections. Barriers significantly decrease exposure to the organism itself, in the vagina with the condom, and at the cervix with the diaphragm and cervical cap. Decreased exposure not only means a lower *rate* of exposure; it also means—especially when the condom is used—a smaller absolute number of organisms, which gives the body a fighting chance to ward off infection. (A diaphragm should be left in for at least 6 hours after coitus, but please, remember to remove it after that).

Contraceptive creams, jellies, and foams are not only spermicidal (and some organisms attach themselves to the sperm itself); they also have bactericidal and viricidal properties. Furthermore, foam is *always* available—as are condoms—over the counter, even on the spur of the moment.

You protect yourself if you use a diaphragm and/or a spermicidal substance. You protect yourself *and* your partner if *he* uses a condom. **If you engage in casual sexual encounters, use a condom . . . for both your sakes.** (There is no reason why you should not carry a good brand of condom yourself.) **Any man who refuses to wear a condom** *if you ask him to* **is not worth going to bed with: he doesn't care very much about himself, and cares less about you.**

When You Go to the Doctor

- Don't douche beforehand. Daintiness is not the issue; correct diagnosis is.
- Make sure the doctor does a wet-mount smear . . . and ask to see the slide yourself. Clinical judgment is not enough; the most s/he can say from observation of the vagina itself is that it "looks like" trich, or candida, or whatever. The wet-mount is the doctor's most useful diagnostic tool; a culture should be a fall-back in most cases, used where there is some question of multiple organisms, or where an infection proves difficult to treat. What's more, a wet-mount is free, and cultures can be expensive.
- Don't get a blitz treatment for vaginitis or cervicitis. It is *your* responsibility to find out—as well as your doctor's—*exactly* what you have.
- Sexually active women should *request* regular testing for sexual infections (you *must* not count on your doctor to suggest them, or even do them routinely) on the following schedule:)
  every 3 months: **gonorrhea culture**
                                   wet-mount for vaginitis
  every 6 months: **VDRL for syphilis**
                                   Pap smear for cervical changes

Even women who have a single consistent sexual partner should play it safe and have all this done once a year—especially the Pap test. (See the next section, If You Are Pregnant, for a special schedule.)

If You Are Pregnant

It's bad enough if *you* have a sexual infection; for your baby it can be devastating . . . or lethal. The damage that sexual infections do to infants is epidemic, and perhaps the greatest tragedy associated with the irresponsibility of the sexually active.

This year, almost <u>50,000</u> babies will suffer the effects of a sexual infection transmitted to them by their mothers. Nearly 10,000 will die almost immediately and another 10,000 will suffer the lifelong effects of the infection, including brain damage and mental retardation (often severe enough that the child will have to be institutionalized until it dies), blindness, deafness, and physical deformity. Many of the rest will have local or systemic disease and birth defects that will make the first months of their lives a horror. (See the chart on pp. 164–165.)

The dreadful irony is that in almost every case, these 50,000 little babies need not have suffered; that pregnant women pay so much attention to the threat of German measles, avoidance of drugs, and correct diet, and so little to the effects of having a sexual infection during pregnancy and at the time of birth, is only one more instance of our inability to be realistic about our responsibilities as sexually liberated people. It is sure that if any *other* condition were causing this rate of death and illness in the infant population, there would be great outcry and immediate attempts to eradicate the health problem.

INFECTIONS TO TEST FOR

Sexual infections that you will want to be tested—and if necessary treated—for (in general order of their capacity to do damage) are:

- **Group B streptococcus,** which can cause (frequently lethal) meningitis and respiratory distress in newborns. The organ-

160

ism *may* be sexually transmitted (although some studies have found its presence unrelated to sexual practices), and seems to be part of the normal vaginal—as well as mouth and intestinal—flora in *some* women. Nearly 15,000 new-borns a year contract this disease . . . and the death rate is high. One third of women with gonorrhea also have Group B strep.

- **herpes simplex virus,** usually transmitted during vaginal de-livery by an infected mother (HSV-2) but also from oral le-sions after birth. Babies have inadequate immune defenses to herpesviruses, and a case of HSV is often fatal. (See HSV section in Part II for further information.)
- **cytomegalovirus,** a fairly innocuous and usually asympto-matic condition in adults which is devastating to infants and is transmitted from an infected mother *in utero, probably* through the placenta, but possibly from ascending vaginal infection. 10% of women have CMV on their cervices. 25% of all seriously retarded newborns have congenital CMV, and it is the most common *viral* cause of brain damage—even more than German measles (rubella)—in babies. Though it is hard to know for sure, it is thought that CMV damages as many as 10,000 babies a year . . . which represents a small proportion of those babies who actually may have been ex-posed to it, and excrete virus, or form antibodies to it.
- **syphilis,** a particularly horrifying (because of the high rate of physical deformities in survivors) and totally avoidable dis-ease. Effects of congenital syphilis may not manifest them-selves until much later in a child's—or even an adult's—development, and the list of potential problems is long and gruesome. Maternal syphilis infects the baby *in utero:* If the mother is treated before the 4th month of gestation, the baby will not have the disease; and if she is treated later, the baby can be cured before it is born . . . and, one hopes, before it is damaged. (See the discussion on syphilis in Part II.)
- **chlamydia trachomatis,** the organism responsible for most of the infectious blindness in the world (trachoma), con-tracted when the baby passes through an infected birth canal. Chlamydia also causes a pneumonia-like disease in newborns and is associated with prematurity. A new mother who already has chlamydia is at much higher risk for child-

161

birth (puerperal) fever; almost one third of mothers with chlamydial infections during pregnancy will develop it.

- **gonorrhea,** which causes gonorrheal conjunctivitis in babies who catch it from an infected mother, and can result in blindness. The good news is that babies born in hospitals are routinely treated to prevent gonorrheal conjunctivitis.
- **warts,** which can be picked up from the maternal genital tract and may cause upper respiratory tract lesions in babies. The lesions can interfere with breathing, swallowing, and—eventually—talking.
- **candida,** which is not serious, but inasmuch as a pregnant woman develops this fungal overgrowth as much as twenty times as frequently as a nonpregnant one, a woman should be aware that, passed to her baby during vaginal delivery, it can manifest itself in an oral infection called thrush that interferes with nursing. It can also cause a rash in the diaper area.

TESTING SCHEDULE FOR SEXUAL INFECTIONS

As soon as you know you are pregnant you should be tested for

> **gonorrhea** (by culture)
> **syphilis** (by blood test: VDRL)
> (Chlamydia should be added to this list as soon as culture techniques are widely available.)

If you have

> **recurrent genital herpes,** you will want to be cultured now to establish a baseline count of possible asymptomatic viral shedding. If your partner has recurrent HSV-2, you will want to know whether you also have it.

In the fourth or fifth month you should repeat the above tests if you have reason to think you may have been exposed—even before you were pregnant—to one of these infections. You may also want to be tested at this time for

> **CMV,** which is very difficult to diagnose. However, if one is very suspicious, cultures can be obtained and antibody levels may be useful. Even if cultures are positive, the baby may still not be affected.

At the beginning of the last month you should repeat the tests for

gonorrhea
syphilis
herpes

and then continue to be cultured for **herpes** once a week until delivery. (Your doctor will have certain management decisions to make if your herpes enters the active stage, or if you commonly have asymptomatic shedding.)

And add a test for

Group B streptococcus

Presumably both

warts

and

candida

will have typical clinical signs.

TREATMENT WHEN YOU ARE PREGNANT

Always tell a doctor that you are pregnant (even if you only suspect it) before taking *anything* s/he prescribes. If you are not being treated by a gynecologist it may not occur to a doctor to ask, and there are some drugs you do not want to be taking when you are pregnant. Among them are

- some antibiotics (especially tetracycline, which stains babies' teeth)
- Flagyl (metronidazole)
- some anti-fungal agents
- podophyllin (used against warts)
- bug-killers like Kwell

Where treatment is concerned, it is much easier to treat a mother for a vaginal—or in the case of syphilis, a systemic—infection than to treat a newborn . . . and indeed, some of these infections become almost *un*treatable once the baby has them. A mother can be treated right up until the time of delivery; the mucus plug in the cervix in most cases protects the baby from vaginal infection until then. It is almost never too late to be tested *and* treated.

SEXUAL INFECTIONS THAT THREATEN BABIES
(all figures approximate)

INFECTIONS	DISEASE CAUSED IN THE INFANT	APPROX-IMATE NUMBER OF TRANS-MISSIONS PER YEAR THAT HARM BABIES	SYMPTOMS IN MOTHER	ROUTE OF INFECTIO
group B streptococcus	streptococcal meningitis	15,000	vaginitis (rare)	vaginal
cytomegalo-virus (CMV)	cytomegalic inclusion disease	up to 10,000 (represents 10% disease rate after infection)	10% have mono-nucleosis-like disease	probably placental
herpes simplex virus (HSV-1) (HSV-2)	HSV	50% of infants born to women with *active* HSV-2 (perhaps 1,000)	see HSV, pp. 86, 93, and 97	oral (HSV-1) cervical/vul (HSV-2)
syphilis	congenital syphilis		see syphilis, p. 60 (often none)	placental
chlamydia	chlamydial infection	No data for U.S.	often none (see chlamydia, p. 71)	genital tract
gonorrhea	gonorrheal conjunctivitis		often none (see gonorrhea, p. 50)	cervical

		MAJOR EFFECTS OF SEXUAL INFECTIONS ON BABIES	
•EATH/ STILL- BIRTH	**BRAIN DAMAGE & RETAR- DATION**	**OTHER PROBLEMS**	**CURE FOR BABIES**
50%	25%	Remaining 25% may suffer from blindness, deafness, pneumonia or breathing difficulties or other systemic diseases	sensitive to penicillin but hard to cure in infants
	30%	All affected infants at risk for blindness and/ or deafness	none
0–60%	25%	25% will survive systemic disease	systemic antivirals may lessen effects of disease
30%	All *surviving* infants at high risk for physical deformity and organ involvement		none for deformities; penicillin
known	unknown but probably signif- icant	In *surviving* infants, 50% chance of chlamydial conjunctivitis (trachoma), the most common infectious cause of blindness in the world, affecting some 500 million individuals. 10% chance of pneumonia or breathing difficulties	antibiotics
◄ pli- ble	not appli- cable	Can cause blindness in untreated infants	silvernitrate solution

165

A WORD ABOUT PREGNANCY ITSELF

If there is an epidemic of sexual infections, there is a mega-epidemic of unwanted pregnancies.

Pregnancy itself is a health hazard. So is abortion. What happens to you while you are pregnant and after giving birth—or as a consequence of termination of a pregnancy—may have serious consequences for your future fertility and capacity to bear children, your general health, and even your life. And the emotional, physical, and psychological effects on a child born to a woman (a girl who is pregnant *is* a woman, whatever her age) who did not intend to have him or her, and cannot play the roles of responsible provider, teacher, and devoted parent, is a child at much greater risk than from all the sexual infections and their effects put together.

Healthy sex is responsible sex, and there is a big difference between procreation and recreation. If you *really* don't want to take foolish chances with your health, don't get pregnant before you are prepared, willing, and responsible enough. You will be hurting more people than just yourself.

FOR MEN

*being responsible • symptoms of sexual infection in men • general
categories of male infections • signs of trouble in a female
partner • protecting yourself and protecting your
partner • contraception*

Men are more fortunate than women when it comes to sexual
infections in that they are more likely to have noticeable symptoms if they have caught something . . . which means they can
get themselves treated before a minor infection becomes a major
problem that threatens fertility, general health, and even one's
life.

Men are also less shy in their dealings with their own bodies.
They are more familiar with their genitals—used to handling and
seeing them—and more alert to suspicious changes. Having a
sexual infection is considerably less traumatic for a man than for
a woman; indeed, in many sectors of our culture, having the clap
(gonorrhea) or a case of crabs is almost a rite of passage. For a
woman, such an infection may seem a tragedy.

Being Responsible

Because men and women *do* manifest symptoms of most sexual infections differently, your obligations to a woman with
whom you have a sexual relationship are in some ways heavier—
practically speaking—than the other way around: the first she
may know of an infection she has is when *you* show its symptoms
and tell *her*. Too many men have the attitude "Well, she burned

167

me; let her rot." This is irresponsible at best and brutally murderous at worst; you *must* tell a female partner you suspect is the source of your infection. (See Sexual Etiquette in Part I for graceful ways of imparting such information.) You must also inform any other woman you have had sexual contact with; she may have the infection too and never know it . . . until it is too late.

By the same token, you may also carry an infection from one woman to another without knowing you have done so. Infections like trichomoniasis and *Hemophilus vaginalis* (HV) are often *passed* by men (who become carriers) without their ever knowing it. So if a sex partner says she has an infection that you have no sign of, still consider it an obligation to warn any *other* sex partner that she may have been exposed . . . and then **make sure that everybody in the chain is treated at the same time. This includes you.**

Once more: never *assume* that a woman is aware of having a sexual infection just because you may have caught one from her. And alert any other woman who may have been exposed through contact with you.

Symptoms of Sexual Infection in Men

Symptoms of sexual infection in men are often—although not always—clear-cut. Indications that something is wrong include:

- burning on urination
- discharge from penis
- sores or bumps on or around the genitals . . . even if they don't hurt
- inflammation of the head of the penis or the urethral opening
- swollen glands (lymph nodes) in the groin
- swollen and/or painful testicles
- lower abdominal pain

If you have *any* of these symptoms, you *must* see a doctor who can diagnose the problem. *Sexual infections do not go away unless they are treated,* and you can do considerable damage to yourself—and to other people—if you don't actively seek medical help.

General Categories of Male Infections

URETHRITIS

is inflammation of the mucous membrane lining of the urethra, which can progress to the bladder (cystitis) and may be caused by:

- chlamydia
- gonorrhea
- genital mycoplasmas
- trichomoniasis
- *E. coli* or other coliform bacteria
- HV *(Hemophilus vaginalis)* . . . rarely

Symptoms
- burning on urination
- urethral discharge
- sometimes fever

Chronic urethritis may impair fertility.

EPIDIDYMITIS

is inflammation of the sperm-duct system, which can impair fertility and may be caused by:

- chlamydia (the usual cause in men under 35)
- chronic urinary-tract infection (in men over 35)
- gonorrhea

Symptoms
- feeling of pressure
- pain
- scrotal swelling

Epididymitis doesn't come from "nothing." If you are diagnosed as having this infection, make sure your doctor finds out —and tells you—what has *caused* it . . . or you put yourself at risk for reinfection from a female partner who is carrying the organism.

PROSTATITIS

is inflammation of the prostate gland, which circles the urethra like a doughnut and produces most of the material of semen (of which sperm itself is only a small part). Prostatitis may be a complex of problems that is either of infectious *or* noninfectious origin, but only a doctor can tell what is causing it. Noninfectious prostatitis is not well understood.

Some Infectious Causes of Prostatitis
- genital mycoplasmas
- gonorrhea
- trichomoniasis
- staphylococcus
- streptococcus

Some Noninfectious Causes of Prostatitis
- old age
- irritation of the prostate because of too much sudden—or too little regular—sexual activity

Symptoms
- slight discharge
- a feeling of fullness
- urinary discomfort, urgency, and frequency
- ejaculation can temporarily relieve symptoms

THINGS *NOT* TO WORRY ABOUT

- **penile papules,** pearly bumps usually found around the head of the penis. They are enlarged sebaceous glands, and are neither harmful nor infectious. (Do make sure, however, that they are not venereal warts.)
- **jock itch** (*tinea cruris;* see discussion of this in Part II). There is not much you can do about jock itch once you have contracted it because it is very difficult to get rid of completely and is likely to recur whenever conditions (warmth, wetness, and friction) are right. If you are prone to jock itch, you should be especially careful about cleanliness, about drying yourself thoroughly after bathing, and about wearing absorbent underclothing that does not bind or rub.

Any man with recurrent jock itch should remember that he *can* give it to his female partner; it is a communicable fungus . . . and consequently a sexually transmitted infection.
- **venous congestion,** which can cause priapism (prolonged erection) or "blue balls." In *rare* cases such congestion is a sign of trouble. Usually it is a result of trying to maintain an erection without ejaculating.

Signs of Trouble in a Female Partner

It is your responsibility to check out a female partner as best you can in the course of the sex play that usually precedes coitus (this is not intended to interfere with the natural pleasure of exploration and need not be coldly clinical), and while women often seem mysterious and genitally complicated to men, there are some things you can be aware of (*aside* from the fact that many sexual infections in women have no symptoms whatsoever):

- **sores, bumps, and lumps.** It is always safer to assume that any such imperfections are the result of a sexual infection than that they are "nothing." Don't be afraid to ask. You may see or feel something that your female partner has not noticed.

  Sebaceous cysts—small hard lumps under the skin caused by overactive oil glands—as well as occluded hair follicles (and ingrown hairs) *are the exceptions* to the bump rule.

  Remember that some infections manifest themselves on the perineum or around the anus (warts, for example). The looking and touching that is natural in sexual intimacy can be very informative.
- **smell.** It is an unfortunate myth that women are "smelly": any woman who observes good genital hygiene will simply have a characteristic female smell—which should be fresh and clean—just as male semen has a characteristic odor that should not be offensive. A *strong foul* smell is usually an indication of some kind of infection and/or poor hygiene.
- **discharge.** A woman normally has a light, whitish discharge that is a product of the natural cleansing action of the va-

gina. This discharge is to be distinguished from the vaginal lubrication (which may be considerable) that is the result of sexual excitement. Lubrication is slick, colorless (although it may be cloudy), and essentially odorless.

Any heavy, smelly discharge that is opaque or has a sticky and/or lumpy consistency is not a good sign.

A strong fishy odor from the vagina *following* male ejaculation is often an indication of infection by *Hemophilus vaginalis* (HV), which men carry and women get.

Protecting Yourself and Protecting Your Partner

In addition to being observant, there are ways in which you can considerably diminish your chances of either getting a sexual infection or passing one along.

To protect yourself:

• urinate after coitus (urination can wash large numbers of organisms out of the urethra; urine is basically a sterile fluid . . . unless you already have a urinary tract infection).
And

• wash carefully after a sexual encounter. Soap and water go a long way toward keeping you healthy.
And

• don't have sexual intercourse if your penis is already irritated. Too many organisms can set up shop in damaged mucosal tissues.

To protect yourself *and* your partner:

• **Wear a condom:** not 100% sure but damn near. New synthetic materials have made objections to the old "rubbers" obsolete . . . and even an *expensive* condom is cheaper than doctors' bills and prescription drugs.

To protect your partner:

• wash carefully *before* a sexual encounter (this means hands, too).
And

• *always* wash *after* anal intercourse before putting your penis *anywhere* else.

And of course *never* have sex with someone if you know you *have* an infection . . . even if you wear a condom.

Contraception

Since unwanted pregnancies can be considered an epidemic, special care should be taken to prevent pregnancy in a female partner if the two of you do not want a baby. A man *must* share responsibility for birth control.

We bring this up because it is becoming clear that a large number of reproductive-tract infections in women are secondary to post-abortion infection that can leave a woman unable to bear children in the future. In this sense, good sound contraception can be considered doubly prophylactic against sexual infections.

FOR GAY MEN

gays and the "traditional" sexual infections • intestinal infections • AIDS or GRID • viral hepatitis • how and where to get medical care • helping yourself

Homosexual men are suffering a disproportionate amount of the total number of sexual infections, and while numbers can only be extrapolated from public health figures (which means that it is hard to generalize), homosexual men seem to be at much higher risk, not only for catching traditional sexual infections—albeit sometimes in new places—but for creating whole new categories of sexually transmitted disease . . . the intestinal disorders, for instance.

There are reasons for this, and they are directly traceable to two interactive but distinct **factors which distinguish homosexuals epidemiologically** from the heterosexual population (and from gay women):

- typical **homosexual patterns of contact**—what one writer has called "institutionalized promiscuity"—which often means
  a) a greater number of sexual contacts, "limited only," says the same writer, "by the stamina of the participants" . . . and, after all, there is no single factor which puts one more at risk for contracting a sexual infection than the number of sexual contacts, and
  b) among this "active" segment of the homosexual population, the likelihood of the anonymity of the partners,

making an infection difficult—if not impossible—to trace.
- the sexual practices of homosexuals, which almost inevitably include anal eroticism—which can mean
  a) a much higher incidence of sexual infection of the rectum and anus with traditionally "venereal" pathogens,
  b) the frequent occurrence of various types of ano-rectal trauma, and
  c) sexual transmission of intestinal disorders—which until recently were not associated with sexual activity—from anal-oral and anal-genital-oral contact.

Both homosexual patterns *and* practices are implicated in two other health problems of the gay population: AIDS (acquired immune deficiency syndrome), also known as GRID (gay-related immunodeficiency), and viral hepatitis.

Gays and the "Traditional" Sexual Infections

Not only do gay men have their special venereal health problems; they also seem to have more of what ails the rest of us. Here are some statistics (which may or may not be generalizable to the homosexual population as a whole):

- Half of all the men who get syphilis are gay (and men already get syphilis three times as often as women).
- Gay men have a high rate of gonorrhea—especially anal and pharyngeal.
- More than a third of all gay men are likely to have amebiasis . . . a 70-fold increase since 1974.
- Perhaps half of all non-imported intestinal infections are found in gay men.
- Gay men seem to have almost universal CMV (cytomegalovirus; see discussion of CMV in Part II), a herpesvirus implicated in AIDS; the reasons for this are not yet understood.
- Gay men also experience more *recurrences* of EBV (Epstein-Barr virus; see discussion of EBV in Part II)—with more serious consequences—than heterosexuals; the reasons for this are not yet understood.

175

- Viral hepatitis infections—while neither limited to the homosexual population nor transmissible only through sexual contact—have become a significant health problem for homosexuals, who do transmit—and catch—them in this manner.

Most of the "traditional" sexual infections can be passed through a combination of anal-genital-oral contact; those that may manifest themselves anally (proctitis)—as well as genitally, and sometimes orally—are:

- gonorrhea
- syphilis
- chancroid
- chlamydia and LGV (lymphogranuloma venereum)
- HSV-1 and HSV-2 (the herpes simplex viruses)
- venereal warts

In all of the above, lesions (or discharge and inflammation) may be hidden in the rectum. Any pain, itching, or discharge should send you to a doctor immediately . . . and you must *tell* the doctor that you engage in anal-erotic practices, or he will not know what he is looking for.

Intestinal Infections

While heterosexuals whose sexual activities include anal-genital-oral contact are at risk for intestinal infections from these practices, gay men—whose erotic behavior probably focuses on such techniques and almost always includes them—seem to be having an epidemic of infections caused by bacteria, viruses, fungi, protozoa, and worms that are spread through ingestion of fecal matter. (One study determined that a series of men suffering from protozoan infections all had engaged in anilingus; conversely, those who reported no anal-oral contact had no such infections. The route of transmission need not be so direct: Hands, genitals, mouth, and anus can carry organisms or cysts from place to place.)

Gay men are also much more likely to suffer traumatic as well as allergic (from soaps and lubricants) proctitis, and to have what has been referred to as **gay bowel syndrome,** which implies multiple and/or recurrent anogenital infection, trauma, itching, burning, and nonspecific proctitis.

Any change in bowel habits should be investigated by a doctor as soon as possible. Because of the precipitate rise in the occurrence of these enteric infections, most doctors who are used to treating homosexual patients will often take an immediate culture from a gay patient who presents with diarrhea, rather than waiting to see what happens.

AIDS (Acquired Immune Deficiency Syndrome), also known as GRID (Gay-Related Immunodeficiency)

AIDS is not a single disease, but rather a series of potentially fatal conditions associated with a defective immune response, a syndrome—until recently—seen only with congenital and drug-acquired immune deficiencies, or in people otherwise seriously debilitated, and never in "normal" populations. AIDS is especially frightening because it is the first instance of an *acquired* immune disorder (and one that is marked by *greater* immune suppression than when the syndrome is brought on by drugs) that is—apparently—communicable . . . and possibly sexually communicable at that. (It must be stressed, however, that while there are more clues every day as to the genesis and course of the syndrome, very little is known for certain.) Research is difficult not only because of the population involved, but because recognition of the syndrome itself is a problem: AIDS may be silent for a long time, only to "appear" when an associated disease is contracted. ("The period between exposure and the onset of a recognizable illness is not known, but available evidence suggests the average exceeds one year," says one source.)

AIDS has caused something of a panic in the homosexual community, and depending on how it is viewed, there may or may not be justification for such panic. On the one hand, there are still less than 1,000 confirmed cases, and only about 300 deaths. On the other hand, diseases associated with AIDS have killed more people than Legionnaire's disease and toxic shock syndrome combined . . . most of them homosexual or bisexual, although there are other identifiable groups that are also affected: Haitians, intravenous drug abusers, and hemophiliacs (who are perhaps affected through blood transfusions, and for whom it was the second leading cause of death last year). Furthermore, there may be 10 to *100* times as many cases whose symptoms have not yet been identified.

What is especially frightening about this syndrome—beyond its apparent communicability, which is distressing enough on its own—is the odd, often incurable diseases to which AIDS victims are typically prey: Kaposi's sarcoma, a rare skin cancer usually seen only in isolated groups; *Pneumocystis carinii* pneumonia, a particularly lethal pneumonia; and fulminant herpes simplex infections (which is what happens when an HSV infection becomes systemic . . . and potentially lethal). Some AIDS victims get more than one of these diseases, and in fact will develop these (and other strange fungal infections and cancers) one after another until they die from a kind of physical depletion. (40% of the cases of AIDS end in fatalities.) For this reason, any *unusually* persistent viral infection may suggest some immune defect, and should be investigated. **There is as yet no sure cure for any of the diseases associated with AIDS**—although some people are treated with better results than others—but new interventions are being tried all the time.

Here are some things that are known—or thought—about AIDS:

- AIDS *appears* to be communicable. This has been deduced not because some causative agent or organism has been found, but because of what epidemiologists call "clustering," meaning that it occurs in groups of people who have intimate contact with one another . . . although there are clearly factors which predispose one to susceptibility. Clustering has occurred not only in terms of "sexual intimacy chains," but geographically as well, with the large majority of cases (60%) turning up in New York City (in the gay community) and the second largest number appearing in the same community in San Francisco. (The hemophiliac and drug abuse statistics suggest that the responsible factor may be blood-borne.)
- AIDS *may* by associated with CMV (cytomegalovirus, one of

the herpesviruses), although there is no proof. 90% of those who get AIDS have CMV antibodies or active infection. Furthermore, the rate of CMV in the gay population is considerably higher than in the heterosexual population.

- There are other factors which reflect some particularities of the gay lifestyle that *may* interfere with the normal immune response and increase susceptibility to AIDS and/or its associated diseases. Some of these *may* include
  a) certain genetic types
  b) the multiplicity of sexual infections and/or exposure to those infections which can lower resistance. (On average, AIDS victims have had twice as many sex partners as nonvictims.)
  c) the drugs repeatedly taken to cure (b)
  d) the use of certain drugs, popular with gays, to enhance erotic response, especially amyl nitrate, or poppers. (Nitrites—one of the breakdown products of nitrates—are known to suppress immune response.)

SYMPTOMS OF AIDS

are not unlike those of a CMV infection. They may include
- swollen glands
- fever
- general malaise
- achiness
- weight loss

DISEASES ASSOCIATED WITH AIDS

- **Kaposi's sarcoma,** a skin cancer up until now associated with old men of Mediterranean origin, and young black men in Africa.

  Classic Kaposi's is characterized by purplish bumps—which may be either raised or flat, and under the skin or on the surface—on the lower legs and feet (the purple color is because the tumor is vascular, or in cells called squamous cells that originate from blood vessel tissue). The tumors associated with Kaposi's do not "spread" or metastasize; rather, they are what is called multifocal, erupting indepen-

179

dently in a number of places. They may also be internal, found in the lymph nodes (glands), liver, or lungs.

Kaposi's has been treated by excision of the lesions and chemotherapy (including Interferon). The prognosis for a Kaposi's sufferer, however, is far from bright: About a quarter die.

- **Pneumocystis carinii pneumonia,** which is *probably* caused by a fungus (related to the yeasts) which invades and parasitizes lung tissue, causing a pneumonia-like disease. PCP cysts are carried by many animals without harming them, and are possibly inhaled, though the mode of infection is not known for sure.

  As in the case of Kaposi's, before 1980 this disease was known only in people who had congenital or drug-induced immune deficiencies.

  PCP's symptoms include a pneumonia-like shortness of breath, weight loss, diarrhea, fever, and weakness. PCP is not easy to diagnose and less easy to cure: More than half its victims die.

- **fulminant herpes simplex viral infections.** See discussion in HSV section on systemic disease, in Part II.

The first cases of AIDS in heterosexuals who do not fall into one of the above categories are now being reported. It is important to know that *if* AIDS is, in fact, transmissable and/or blood-borne (as the epidemiology suggests) it is only a matter of time until this syndrome—*probably* through bisexual contacts—becomes a health problem for the population at large.

Viral Hepatitis

Hepatitis—or inflammation of the liver—has many causes, and while some of them are secondary effects of other infections, the hepatitis that concerns us—and is more and more considered a sexually transmitted disease (although it is by no means only sexually transmitted)—is viral hepatitis, and is the result of not one but a number of viral infections which share effect (the liver inflammation) and symptoms. Because of both their sexual practices and their patterns, gay men are at higher risk for contracting viral hepatitis than are heterosexuals, and before the advent

of AIDS, hepatitis was considered the most serious of the nonve-
nereal sexually transmitted infections, both because of its capacity to cause debilitating illness and because of its high rate of
complications.

Symptoms of hepatitis range from mild to severe, with a large
number of totally asymptomatic cases (who become "carriers"
of the disease). The mildest symptoms are rather like a low-grade
case of the flu, while symptoms of severer infections may include
fever, nausea and vomiting, jaundice (a yellowing of the skin and
whites of the eyes), and general prostration. If you turn yellow,
you can be pretty sure you have hepatitis. See a doctor immediately.

You should remember that having one type of viral hepatitis
will not protect you from getting another type, although you will
not get the *same* type again. At any rate, a good proportion of us
carry antibodies to at least one type of hepatitis already.

HEPATITIS A (HAV)

also called **infectious hepatitis** or **short-incubation hepatitis,**
accounts for almost three quarters of all cases of viral hepatitis.

This kind of hepatitis is contracted through fecal-oral contami-
nation, which is why gay men have a high rate of HAV. HAV can
also be contracted by eating raw shellfish that has been contaminated by sewage, by drinking polluted water, or from food handled by a hepatitis carrier.

If you have been exposed to HAV, you can protect yourself
from severe infection—and perhaps escape infection altogether
—if you are treated with *immune serum globulin* (called gamma
globulin prophylaxis). This is another reason it is important to
avoid anonymous sexual contacts who cannot let you know—or
whom you cannot inform—that there has been an exposure to
hepatitis.

The incubation period of HAV is from 15 to 45 days (average
25–30).

HEPATITIS B (HBV)

also called **serum hepatitis** or **long-incubation hepatitis,** is
usually spread through blood transfusions or infected needles

(by drug abusers), but as all body fluids (saliva, semen, urine, vaginal and menstrual secretions, in addition to blood) can carry the virus, it is also possible to contract HBV from any kind of intimate contact in which you are exposed to these infected secretions.

While HBV can be caught by anybody, there may be a factor linked to sexual activity that makes gay men a particular target of the infection . . . and indeed, they have much more HBV than do heterosexuals.

The incubation period for HBV is from 50 to 180 days (average 60–90).

HBV has a high rate of asymptomatic carriers.

OTHER VIRAL HEPATITISES

called variously **non-A/non-B,** or **hepatitis C, D,** etc., are, as the name implies, different from HAV and HBV. Little is known about these further kinds of viral hepatitis, except that they are probably not transmitted exclusively by blood transfusions as had been thought, but also possibly by sexual contact.

If you have any signs of hepatitis—and jaundice in particular —you should see a doctor as soon as possible. Secondary hepatitis can also be the result of other sexual infections, such as CMV, EBV, secondary syphilis, or advanced gonorrhea (in women).

How and Where to Get Medical Care

If you are a gay man, you have very specific sex-related health needs, and it can take a measure of sophistication to accurately and adequately diagnose and treat potential problems. Except in those big cities with large homosexual populations, the local health department clinic may not be the right place for you; you want a setting that is well equipped and congenial, with sympathetic personnel who know, for instance, the different varieties of proctitis when they see it, who know when to suspect an intestinal infection, and who are alert to subtler health problems that are *not* specifically venereal but may affect you, like hepatitis and AIDS.

Almost every city with a gay subculture has a network of referrals and/or a health facility catering to that subculture, as well as doctors who are themselves homosexual. Wherever you decide to go, you must feel comfortable enough to be able to be as open and honest as possible about your sexual practices.

Helping Yourself

Good medical care is only *part* of the solution; taking care of yourself requires more of you than simply finding a doctor or a facility (which you should do *before* you think you may have trouble, so that you don't waste time finding somewhere to go) and then being absolutely frank about your sexual practices and contacts . . . although this is a good beginning. You should be tested regularly for sexual infections, be on the lookout for even slight changes in your body or functioning, and be responsible about the number and kind of sexual encounters you engage in.

Because so many of the sexual infections of gay men are in the anus, rectum, and bowel, you should be particularly alert to any itching, swelling, burning or pain, and abdominal cramps, diarrhea, or bloody stools should send you right to your doctor or clinic. You should be regularly examined for anal lesions (warts, syphilis, herpes), and cultured for gonorrhea and intestinal infections. You should also be tested regularly for hepatitis and syphilis (by blood test), as these infections easily can escape detection in gays. And if you begin to have vague feelings of illness, don't hesitate to see a doctor: you may have an active case of CMV or EBV.

The most obvious way of protecting yourself is, of course, to cut down on the number of your sexual contacts . . . and make sure that those you have are not of the "anonymous" variety.

FOR TEENAGERS

special problems of young people • if you think you might have a sexual infection • getting help • staying healthy • contraception— what girls should know • for parents

Here are some statistics that should interest you if you are a teenager . . . or the parent of a teenager:

- **One in seven teens has a venereal disease.**
- 85% of reported venereal disease is in young people aged 15–30.
- Teenagers have especially high rates of gonorrhea, syphilis, and chlamydia, all infections which can compromise reproductive capacity and have serious consequences—because of the likelihood that they will have grave complications— for general health.
- Teenage girls have a high proportion of the PID (pelvic inflammatory disease) which comes from untreated sexual infections (chlamydia and gonorrhea). This also means that **each year perhaps 100,000 young women will have damage done to their reproductive systems** that may make them unable to get pregnant in the future.

Special Problems of Young People

Most young people have not yet come to terms with their sexuality at all . . . much less the threat of a pregnancy or sexual infection. They are embarrassed about sex in general, and while most teens will say they are terrified of getting a sexual infection

—or of getting pregnant—at the same time they often do very little to protect themselves from either. It is not, therefore, just the "new morality" and the sexual freedom of young people that is causing the current problem (although clearly if there were less sexual activity the rate of sexual infection would drop precipitately); it is just as much a combination of embarrassment, fear, ignorance, misinformation, and confusion about what to do or where to go if something is wrong. (You must also, of course, know how to recognize a problem when it arises: the worst place to go for advice or diagnosis is a friend.)

Anybody who is sexually active takes certain risks and must be prepared to deal with the potential consequences of taking those risks. (Teenagers often think of neither risks nor consequences.) If you are old enough to have sex, you are old enough to take responsibility for your sexual activity and—presumably—your sexual pleasure . . . which means, just as it does for an adult, educating yourself, protecting yourself, and taking *immediate* steps to diagnose and treat anything that seems suspicious. You should also be aware that you need not have coitus—sexual intercourse—to contract a sexual infection; kissing, oral-genital contact (15% of the gonorrhea in teenagers, for instance, is pharyngeal—in the throat), and petting (manual stimulation) can spread organisms.

Hesitating to take care of a problem not only can spread your infection to other people; it can also cause serious problems for you in the future that may affect your ability to have children (this is true for men as well as women), your health in general, and even your life.

If You Think You Might Have a Sexual Infection

Frequently teenagers panic if they think they have caught something: they have nightmares of outraged parents, social ostracism, and perpetual ruin and degradation. Unfortunately, rather than catalyzing them to action to protect and/or cure themselves, this panic makes them ignore the "problem" and hope that it will go away: they pretend it just doesn't exist.

Young girls especially often see a sexual infection as cruel and

185

specific punishment for their having been sexually active—which in a way it is, if they have not been responsible in the management of their sex lives—and it certainly *becomes* punishment if a girl waits for a complication like PID to set in . . . in which case she may be "punished" for the rest of her life.

Because it is so distressing for a teen to catch some kind of sexually transmitted disease, and because for many young people such an incident creates long-term emotional disturbances and conflicts about sexuality, <u>it is important for you to think about and prepare for your responsibilities as an adult *before* you engage in adult activities.</u> And this includes thinking about protecting yourself and your partner from unwanted pregnancy as well as from sexual infections . . . not thinking about it later when you are already pregnant or sick. As is true with most "grown-up" activities that teens engage in as a kind of rite of passage into adulthood (such as driving and drinking, as well as exercise of your sexuality), parents are often more uptight about how *responsibly* you initiate yourself into previously forbidden pursuits and pleasures than they are about your actually *doing* them. If you are reading this book, you are probably considering —or are already involved in—a sexual relationship anyway, so the question becomes not whether you do it at all, but whether you know how to take care of yourself and your partner when you *do* do it.

It *is* hard to accept and deal with a possible sexual infection, but it's happened to a lot of kids before you, and, sadly, will happen to many more after you.

If punishment is what you're afraid of, don't forget that people often create their own worst punishments . . . and the punishment in this case is *not* for being a sexual person and exercising your right to pleasure and intimacy; the punishment is for ignorance and irresponsibility.

Getting Help

There is another reason sexual infections among teenagers often go untreated: teens simply do not know what to do. A young person is unlikely to take his/her problem to the friendly old family doctor or pediatrician, both because s/he is embarrassed and ashamed and because of the fear that parents will be told.

If you are like most young people who do not have a private physician they feel close to and can trust, you may feel more comfortable going to a clinic (see the later section, Where to Go for Help, about finding a clinic) where the personnel are used to treating young people like you, and will not make you feel ashamed or dirty. You can go to a health department facility or a Planned Parenthood clinic or affiliate, or you can call the VD Hotline (see Where to Go for Help for numbers), which will put you in touch with a low-cost clinic or private physician in your area.

Contrary to popular opinion, **nowhere does a teenager of any age need a parent's permission to be treated for a sexual infection. (This is not true, by the way, if you are seeking contraceptive advice, which is regulated in different ways in different states . . . although often where laws are in conflict with social concerns, the humanitarian impulse wins out and a clinic will help you anyway. Check with a counselor in the clinic in person. Or call Planned Parenthood for advice.)**

Your privacy is absolutely protected when you are seen in a clinic for a sexual infection. No one will tell your parents. No one will call your home or send incriminating letters. These people aren't concerned with making your life difficult; they want to help you and make sure that you neither pass along your infection nor suffer later consequences from it.

Finally, many clinics—and all health department facilities— are free. And that includes any drugs you may be given. So money is no excuse.

If you still can't figure out where to go, call the Department of Adolescent Medicine at your local hospital and ask for a referral.

The important thing is to get treated. And to get treated immediately. Nothing is "nothing." And nothing goes away by itself.

A last word about getting help: getting help means giving help, so don't think you are protecting a partner by not informing him/ her that you have a sexual infection . . . or by not letting a health facility do the notifying for you. **Protecting a friend means informing a friend.**

Staying Healthy

Now is the time to establish a good relationship with a clinic or doctor—with someone or in some place where you feel comfortable—not later when you are frightened and upset. You can also do yourself a big favor by being tested regularly for sexual infections like gonorrhea and syphilis, because these infections are so frequently asymptomatic. Your health care is your responsibility. It's no longer enough to have that one checkup a year for the school records if you are sexually active.

Contraception—What Girls Should Know

Every young woman must recognize that the contraceptive decisions she makes now—or the lack of them—may affect her fertility for the rest of her life . . . and the most psychologically and physically traumatic decision may be the non-decision of failing to protect herself, getting pregnant, and having an abortion. While abortion is safer than childbirth itself, it is considerably *less* safe than using contraception—*any* contraception—in the first place.

Deciding which contraceptive to use is between you and your doctor, but it is a decision that must not wait: young women have erratic menstrual cycles and for all practical purposes can get pregnant *any* time . . . and all you need is *one* unprotected instance of sexual intercourse to change your life forever. Most teenage girls find that the Pill is the most convenient—and safest—way of protecting themselves, but whatever you choose you must remember that no contraceptive works if it is not used. Some young women are responsible enough to use the diaphragm or cervical cap, so these are an option. An IUD is less likely to be a method of choice for a young girl because not only is an IUD difficult to wear if you have never had a child, but IUDs increase your chance of getting some sexual infections (the bacteria can creep up the cord that hangs into the vagina and enter the uterus).

Fortunately, good contraception, however, is never farther away than the corner drugstore. A condom and contraceptive

foam—used properly and together—offer a very high degree of protection against *both* pregnancy and venereal disease.

So there is no excuse for not protecting yourself. *None.*

For Parents

Sexual activity is a fact of life for most young people, so it is not a question of whether the kids are going to *do* it, but whether they are adequately armed against the consequences of what they *have done* or *are doing* already. Blanket condemnations of teenage sexual activity and punitive attitudes only make the problem worse; until we can be sure of *stopping* premarital sex, we had better concentrate on the results of our having pretended for so long that teenage lives could be regulated in this way. Certainly if there were an epidemic of *airborne* infections among our children that took the same toll as do sexual infections, we would already have done everything in our power to see that the trend was reversed.

Because ignorance and misinformation and fear are so much at the root of the explosion of venereal disease among young people, it is the responsibility of the parents to educate, inform, and encourage a child's sense of responsibility as s/he moves into adulthood . . . to moral precepts certainly, but also to pragmatic considerations. This *can* be done without either encouraging sexual activity—even tacitly—or terrifying a child into withdrawal or rebellion . . . and *without* invading his/her privacy.

A calm, rational, nonjudgmental discussion of some of the risks and consequences of being sexually active should be as much a part of an eventual parent-child talk on sex as should an encouragement of the child to consider the magnitude of the step taken—and the power of sexuality itself. If our children are afraid to turn to their parents—to ask their opinions and support —whom will they turn to? And what will this lack of communication cost them? And us?

One must, in the end, subscribe to the Daredevil's Theory of Progress: when something doesn't work out in spite of careful planning—when the motorcycle falls into the Snake River Canyon, or the car fails to make the jump over twelve flaming buses —there is only one thing you can know for sure: whatever you did last time doesn't work, so don't do *that* again. Our old attitudes have accomplished nothing . . . or perhaps made the problem of teenage venereal disease worse. (Certainly it *is* worse, and who is to blame?) If we love our children we must find some way to help them, and to teach them to take care of themselves . . . even if we don't approve of all their behavior.

The health and well-being of our children is a high price to pay for parental self-righteousness and moral rigidity.

WHERE TO GO FOR HELP

If you think you may have a sexual infection, you have—in most areas of this country—*at least* four choices of where to go for diagnosis and treatment:

- private physician
- the health department (public health clinics)
- Planned Parenthood and affiliated clinics
- hospital venereal disease clinics and free-standing clinics

You would think that with this many choices, *no one* would let a sexual infection go undiagnosed and untreated. If you are bewildered and don't know where to start or whom to call, you may want to begin by telephoning the

VD NATIONAL HOTLINE

This is a program of the American Social Health Association (ASHA). It has trained volunteers to answer your questions over the phone and refer you to any of the above facilities—or doctors—in your area. The Hotline operates from 8 A.M. to 8 P.M. Pacific Standard Time from Monday to Friday, 10 to 6 on weekends.

The **toll-free** number is
800–227–8922
800–982–5883 in California

The address of the people who run the Hotline is
260 Sheridan Avenue
Palo Alto, CA 94306

The Hotline is supported jointly by the U.S. Centers for Disease Control and the ASHA. The Hotline gets more than 300 calls a day, and the people who answer the phones are trained to give you whatever comfort and information you may need. (There is also a quarterly newsletter, *The Hotliner*.)

ASHA also runs the Herpes Resource Center (see discussion of Herpes simplex virus in Part II).

PRIVATE PHYSICIANS

Most women already have a doctor who specializes in problems of the reproductive and genital tracts (a gynecologist), so they have someone with whom they have established a relationship to consult if they think they may have contracted a sexual infection.

Men, on the other hand, usually do not have analogous medical care (a urologist) unless they have had serious problems of the reproductive or urinary tract that have required the attentions of a specialist. If a man goes to his dermatologist, internist, or family physician for the diagnosis, he should realize that all doctors are not necessarily trained to diagnose a sexual infection, and that the kindly old family standby may not have seen a syphilis chancre since medical school. For this reason, some men find it most efficient to go directly to a clinic for diagnosis of a venereal problem, even if they have a private doctor.

CLINICS: PUBLIC HEALTH SERVICE, HOSPITALS, FREE-STANDING CLINICS

Men are usually more comfortable in clinics than women, and it *can* be more than disconcerting to find yourself in a large room lined up with lots of other people . . . all of whom are there for the same reasons you are. However, clinics are in most cases extremely efficient and have the advantage of
- having already seen anything *you* might have;
- sympathetic personnel who have heard it all before;
- equipment and diagnostic techniques that you are unlikely

to find in even the best-equipped doctor's office . . . and that
may bring you to a big clinic sooner or later anyway; and

- **they are either low-cost or free . . . including medication.**

Health Department clinics are also anxious to help you notify
anyone else who may have been exposed, and will do it in a way
that neither implicates you nor violates the privacy of the person
notified. Health departments are very strict about confidentiality:
not even a court order will release your records. (The New York
City Health Department sends out innocuous-looking letters to
your contacts—coded in a way that tells *them* but no one else,
including the recipient, what s/he is being notified for—but simply says that s/he has an appointment at such-and-such a time at
such-and-such an address and giving a number to call for further
information. It is the rare person who will not call to inquire
about the letter.)

Health department personnel respond to any questions with a
kind, supportive attitude, like "We're worried about you." They
really do care.

**A note about notifying partners: whether *you* do it, or the
health department does it, it must be done by someone.** Sometimes people think they are protecting a partner by withholding
his/her name, but just the opposite is true. If you *really* want to
protect a partner, *inform* him/her . . . or allow the health department to do it anonymously.

Health departments do have some limitations: They are often
not really equipped to diagnose and manage more complicated
—and subtler—conditions . . . viral hepatitis, for instance, or epididymitis, or PID and endometriosis, or the problems of babies
who have been infected with sexually transmitted diseases.
Some health departments only treat the old-line venereal diseases and will send you somewhere else for bladder problems,
or intestinal infections, or skin problems. You must just check
and see, and then pursue the best medical care for yourself.

**A teenager does not need parental approval to be treated for
a sexual infection. And your parents will not be told.**

PLANNED PARENTHOOD AND AFFILIATES

Women may want to go to a Planned Parenthood clinic or one
of their affiliates, of which there are 190 in forty-two states and

Washington, D.C. If you want to find the local PP representative, you can either look in the phone book (they all have "Planned Parenthood" somewhere in their names), or call the Planned Parenthood National Headquarters in New York at 212-541-7800 and ask for the closest facility. <u>Planned Parenthood is an absolutely reliable source for information, service, and referral ... both for the diagnosis and treatment of sexual infections, and for contraception.</u>

The time to think about good medical care is not, however, when you suspect you have a problem; the time to connect with a clinic or a doctor you like and trust is *before* something happens. And of course, if you are sexually active, you are going to want to make sure that you are completely checked out for infections every few months. (See the next section, Staying Healthy.)

The point is to be diagnosed and treated, however you want to accomplish this. Go where you are most comfortable. But **go** when you have a problem, and see your medical advisers regularly even if you do not.

STAYING HEALTHY

or DON'T JUST COUNT ON YOUR DOCTOR

Staying healthy is really a four-point program:

- **prevention**
- **regular checkups**
- **knowing the signs of trouble**
- **getting *immediate* medical care if something is amiss**

And, of course, being responsible and
notifying any partners of exposure to a sexual infection

PREVENTION

It is a sad truism that in this country we are more often focused on cure than on prevention. If only we could teach health, concern with cure would be secondary. There are a number of things you can do to diminish the risk of ever *catching* a sexual infection:

- Know what to look for in a partner that may indicate the presence of an infection . . . and *look.*
- Use a **barrier method of contraception:** the **condom,** the **diaphragm with spermicidal cream or jelly,** or either of these with **contraceptive foam.** Every layer of material between you and a partner is a layer of protection. (Spermicidal substances are often bactericidal and viricidal as well.) Condoms and foam can be bought at any drugstore.
- Keep clean. Soap and water can still work wonders, especially for the uncircumcised male. Women should of course keep the vulva and perineum clean, but must be cautious

about douching. (See For Women.) And <u>keep your hands clean.</u> Unless touching is not part of your sexual repertoire.

- Don't ask for trouble by using "sexual aids" that may have been used previously by someone else (vibrators, for instance). Women should not share douching equipment. Any lubricants should be water-soluble. (This means sterile surgical jellies, for instance, rather than Vaseline.) And don't use implements for sexual stimulation that can abrade, scratch, or otherwise irritate delicate tissue. Anything that touches mucous membrane must be scrupulously clean. In other words, don't let it touch mucous membrane if you wouldn't put it in your mouth.
- <u>Urinate after coitus.</u> This is smart for both men *and* women. Urine is essentially sterile, and a good stream can wash pathogens out of the urinary tract.
- Of course, you could always just stop having sex. . . .

REGULAR CHECKUPS

If the general public is reluctant to educate itself about sexual infections, so are the people who are in charge of our health: inadequate routine screening, careless diagnosis, and ineffective treatment—often without followup—account at least partly for the current epidemic of sexual infections. In defense of the doctors, however, medical care must be a partnership; what the patient doesn't expect and/or demand, the doctor may be hesitant to bring up.

Doctors are, for the most part (except for those who work in inner cities, or clinics specializing in sexual infections), no less uncomfortable with the topic of sexual infection than are patients. They may be reluctant to suggest routine screenings for fear of insulting you, and many doctors in general practice do not keep up on the latest information on the diagnosis and treatment of sexual infections. <u>It is up to *you* to ask for regular testing,</u> and to know something about which tests are appropriate. It is up to *you* to be honest about the kind—and level—of sexual activity you engage in. And if you are not comfortable enough with your present medical care to be forthcoming and ask for the kind of monitoring which is so important to your health if you are a sexually active person, find someone/someplace where you *are* comfortable . . . and be seen *regularly,* on a reasonable schedule for the maintenance of *your* health.

If you are sexually active, you should—at least—have a VDRL (blood test) for syphilis every 6 months, and a culture for gonorrhea every 3 months. (Chlamydia testing is still in a primitive stage, and cost prohibits its being done routinely.) In addition, women should have a wet-mount smear to check for organisms in the vagina every 3 months. (See the section For Women for a more complete schedule, and the section If You Are Pregnant within that section for a pregnancy schedule.) Often you must *ask* for these tests; many doctors do not routinely suggest them. If you are concerned about money, remember that **public health service or health department clinics test for these infections for free.** (See separate sections for special health considerations.)

And never let a doctor put you off with "It's nothing," or "Let's wait a few days to see if it clears up." It is *much more likely than not* that if you *have* a suspicious symptom, you have an infection that is causing it. Many infections are best diagnosed when they are active and visible—before they "clear up" (which can just as well mean that they have evolved into a phase of more serious complications). If you value your sexual health—as well as your health in general—you will make it your business to have your fears allayed . . . or your infection cured.

KNOWING THE SIGNS OF TROUBLE

Your first line of defense is knowledge, the kind of knowledge that alerts you to a problem before it wreaks havoc. How often it happens that someone "just didn't *notice*" a fairly classic symptom . . . or ignored it because s/he had little idea of the implications of the failure to treat a sexual infection!

With good information available, there is no excuse for "missing" the first signs of trouble; the time to educate yourself to all the things you never wanted to know about sex is not when you get sick, but *before.* Being sexually active *always* carries the risk of possible infection—*no one* is immune, regardless of socioeconomic level, education, or sexual habits—so perhaps knowing in advance what to watch for is not unlike being required to learn the laws of the road before getting behind the wheel.

GETTING IMMEDIATE MEDICAL CARE IF SOMETHING IS AMISS

Don't wait. And if you *do* have a sexual infection, don't wait to tell your partner(s) . . . after all, you got this from *somewhere,* and may have passed it along before you even knew you were infected yourself.

We hope you have a doctor or clinic already. If you don't, you should. (See the preceding section, Where to Go for Help.)

In the end, staying healthy is *your* business, not just your doctor's.

GLOSSARY

AIDS acronym for "acquired immune deficiency syndrome; a phenomenon recently increasingly seen among gay men. Also known as GRID ("gay-related immune deficiency").

amebiasis intestinal infection caused by amoebas, which are single-celled organisms. May be sexually transmitted.

amenorrhea absence of menstruation

anal eroticism stimulation of the anus for sexual pleasure. This practice has created a whole new subgroup of sexually transmitted infections.

anilingus oral stimulation of the anus

apthous (*ap*-thus) lesions *inside* the mouth which are sometimes mistaken for recurrent HSV-1 (oral herpes). Little is known about apthous.

asymptomatic having no apparent symptoms—which is not the same as having no infection

auto-inoculation infection of oneself

barrier contraception methods of contraception which help prevent exposure to sexual infections as well. They include the condom, the diaphragm, and spermicidal foams and jellies.

Bartholin's glands two tiny glands located on either side of the entrance to the vagina. These glands can sometimes become infected by bacteria.

Betadine a brown antiseptic solution used in surgery and sometimes for douching

blitz treatment getting a broad-spectrum antibiotic (meant to cure many things) to cure a "nonspecific" infection or combination of infections. Not always a good idea.

blue balls swelling and pain in the testicles from chronic sexual arousal without the release of ejaculation. The parallel in women is pelvic congestion.

bubo (*boo*-boe) inflamed swelling of the lymph nodes, especially in the groin

candidiasis infection by *Candida albicans,* a yeastlike fungus. Sometimes called moniliasis *(Monilia),* or just "a yeast infection."

carcinoma a kind of cancer; a tumor of the skin, mucous membranes, or glands

cervical cap a barrier method of contraception—not widely, but increasingly, used. A cap of rubber, synthetic material, or even silver fits over the cervix tightly and stays in place by mild suction. A cervical cap is smaller than a diaphragm.

cervix (*sir*-vix) literally, neck. The lower end of the uterus, which protrudes—and opens—into the vagina. Sperm ascend through the opening (called the os) to fertilize an egg. Menstrual fluid also comes through the os, and infection can get up into the uterus through it. **Cervicitis** is inflammation of the cervix

chancre (*shank*-er) a sore or ulcer in the genital region, usually associated with syphilis, but also with chancroid

chancroid (*shank*-royd) a sexually transmitted bacterial infection

chlamydia (kla-*mi*-di-a) shorthand for *Chlamydia trachomatis,* an intermediate organism which causes many sexual—and other—infections

circumcision surgical removal of the foreskin of the penis, exposing the glans, or head (usually done on infants)

clap slang for gonorrhea

clitoris (*kli*-tor-is) a highly sensitive organ and the site of intense pleasure for a woman when it is stimulated. The clitoris develops from the same tissue that forms the penis in the male; indeed, if it is examined closely, it *looks* like a tiny, half-buried penis.

CMV cytomegalovirus, a herpesvirus responsible for a quarter of serious infant retardation

coitus (*ko*-i-tus) sexual intercourse between a man and a woman—i.e., a penis in a vagina

condom (*kon*-dum) a sheath made of thin material—rubber, a synthetic, or sheep gut—that fits over the penis and prevents semen from being deposited in the vagina. It also helps protect both partners from exposure to disease. Also called a *rubber* or a *prophylactic.*

congenital existing at birth. A congenital condition may or may not be inherited.

contraception the use of barriers, drugs, or abortifacients (which prevent implantation of a fertilized egg, e.g., the IUD) to prevent pregnancy. There are also nonartificial means of contraception —"rhythm" and withdrawal (*coitus interruptus*)—which are less often reliable. New methods, like the examination of cervical mucus, are being perfected and show much promise.

Cowper's glands a pair of glands in the male near the prostate. During sexual excitement they secrete small amounts of mucus-like fluid that probably neutralizes any anti-sperm climate in the urethra and is one component of seminal fluid.

crabs pubic lice

culture in medicine, a living sample of a microorganism, deliberately grown in controlled conditions so that it can be identified

cunnilingus (kun-i-*ling*-gus) oral stimulation of the vulva

cystitis (sis-*tie*-tis) inflammation of the bladder. Symptoms may be pain or burning on urination, or a feeling of fullness or urgency. Both men and women get cystitis.

diaphragm a dome-shaped contraceptive device, made of rubber or a synthetic material, that is worn internally by a woman and fits over the cervix

dose slang for gonorrhea, as in "catch a dose"

douche (doosh) washing the vagina with a stream of water under pressure

dysmenorrhea painful menstruation

dyspareunia painful intercourse, *sometimes* as a result of a sexual infection

EBV Epstein-Barr virus, one of the herpesviruses and a frequent cause of infectious mononucleosis

ectopic literally, out of place. In an ectopic pregnancy, the embryo develops outside the uterus, usually in a fallopian tube. Ectopic pregnancies can cause hemorrhage and even death. They are more likely to occur when there is scar tissue in the tubes from a prior infection that has spread.

ejaculation the expulsion of semen during orgasm

endometrium the mucous membrane that lines the uterus and sloughs off during menstruation. **Endometriosis** is the presence of this tissue in the pelvic cavity.

epidemiology the study of patterns of disease in a population, especially epidemics

epididymis the network of tubules in the scrotum that connects the sperm ducts to the testicles. **Epididymitis** is inflammation of the epididymis, usually caused by chlamydia.

fallopian tubes tubes through which an egg passes on its way from the ovary to the uterus. Fertilization takes place in the tube.

fellatio (fe-*lay*-she-o) oral stimulation of the penis

fetus the unborn child after the second month of pregnancy. It is called an embryo before then.

flora plant life. The flora, or microflora, of the vagina is the bacteria, fungi, and other organisms that grow there.

foams contraceptive method in which foaming substances in the vagina act as a barrier to sperm. Foams also have bactericidal and viricidal properties.

follicle any small sac or gland for secretion or excretion, as a hair follicle or ovarian follicle

foreskin in males, the skin covering the end of the penis. This is what is surgically removed during circumcision. It is also called the prepuce. (Women also have a "foreskin" on the clitoris, called the clitoral hood.)

fungus a plantlike organism

genital mycoplasmas intermediate organisms that can cause sexual infection

giardiasis an intestinal infection caused by protozoa and sometimes sexually transmitted

glans the sensitive head of the penis or the clitoris

gonorrhea a sexually transmitted bacterial infection

granuloma inguinale a sexually transmitted bacterial infection

GRID an acronym for Gay-Related Immune Deficiency. Also known as AIDS.

gynecologist a doctor who specializes in the treatment of problems of the female reproductive tract

healthy sex responsible sex

herpes the common but inaccurate name for HSV-2, or genital herpes. The herpesvirus family is large.

HV *Hemophilus vaginalis,* a bacterium, or the infection, usually of the vagina, that it causes

hymen a crescent-shaped fold of skin that protects the vaginal entrance (introitus) in a girl or woman who has not had it broken either because of sexual or strenuous physical activity

impotence the inability of a man to get or sustain an erection. Don't confuse it with infertility.

incubation period the time it takes for the symptoms of an infection to appear

infertility lack of ability to produce offspring

inflammation reaction of the body to injury or irritation, characterized by pus, redness, and pain

inguinal (*in*-gwi-nel) pertaining to the groin

inoculate infect

introitus (in-*troy*-tus) opening, as in vaginal introitus

-itis a suffix meaning inflammation. For example, vaginitis is inflammation of the vagina.

IUD acronym for "intrauterine device," a plastic or metal device which is inserted in the uterus and *may* work by preventing the fertilized egg from implanting itself in the uterine wall

jellies or jels, or gels. Used for contraception and/or lubrication.

They should be nongreasy and water-soluble (i.e, *not* Vaseline). They may have spermicidal properties.

jock itch   a sexually communicable fungus infection of the genital area. Also called *tinea cruris.*

labia   (*lay*-bee-a) the lips of the vagina. The **labia majora** are the outer lips; the **labia minora** are the smaller inner lips.

lesion   an injury, sometimes as the result of infection, but not necessarily

leukorrhea   (lou-kor-*ree*-a) a normal, whitish discharge from the vagina

LGV   lymphogranuloma venereum, a complication of a chlamydial infection.

masking   when one condition hides another by obscuring its symptoms

meatus   (me-*ay*-tis) opening, for instance the urethral meatus in the penis

menarche   the onset of menstruation

molluscum contagiosum   a viral infection that can be sexually transmitted

mucosa; mucous membrane   thin surface tissue which is moist from constant secretion of mucus. Mucous membranes are found at the junctures of the inside and outside of the body and are especially susceptible to infection. The vagina, vulva, penis, lips, and anus are all covered with mucous membrane. The cervix, urethra, rectum, mouth, throat, and eyes are covered with mucus-*secreting* membranes.   Some infections are particular to mucus-secreting membranes, and some to mucous membranes.

necrotic   dead or dying; said of tissue destroyed by an infection

neonate   a newborn baby

os   opening or orifice, as in the os of the cervix

ovaries   female sex glands (gonads) in which eggs (ova) that are released every month are stored

ovulation   the release of the ovum from a follicle on the surface of the ovary

papules (penile)   pearly bumps, usually around the head of the penis, that are harmless

pathogen   any organism that causes a disease

pediculosis pubis   skin irritation caused by the bite of pubic lice

perineum   the area between the vaginal entrance and the anus in a woman, and between the scrotum and the anus in a man

peritoneum   the strong transparent membrane that contains the intestines. **Peritonitis** is inflammation of the peritoneum, sometimes caused by the spread of a sexual infection.

pH   symbol used to express the degree of acidity or alkalinity of a substance. pH values run from 0 to 14, with 7 the neutral point;

values of less than 7 are increasingly acidic as they approach 0, and values of more than 7 are increasingly alkaline as they approach 14.

ping-pong effect when sexual partners pass a sexual infection back and forth between them because they have not been treated at the same time

pinworms an intestinal infestation most common among children

placenta the organ that develops on the wall of the uterus during pregnancy at the site of the implantation of the fertilized egg. It is expelled after the child is born and is thus also called the afterbirth. The placenta nourishes the fetus (to which it is attached by the umbilical cord) and carries away waste material. It protects the fetus against many, but not all, of the substances in the mother's body, including drugs and infections. Infections which cross the so-called **placental barrier**—like syphilis and CMV—can do great damage to the developing baby, as can drugs taken by the mother.

proctitis inflammation of the rectum and/or anus

proctologist doctor who specializes in diseases of the rectum and anus

prophylactic anything used to prevent or protect against disease. Also refers to a condom, which does just that.

prostate gland a doughnut-shaped organ around the neck of the bladder in the male which supplies one of the components of semen, called prostatic fluid. **Prostatitis** is inflammation of the prostate; it is a common problem in men after middle age and does not *necessarily* result from an infection.

protozoa microscopic single-cell animals which can sometimes cause infections in human beings

pus yellowish-white sticky fluid produced when white blood cells rush to the site of an infection to isolate and destroy invading microorganisms so that the body can repair itself. Pus is made up of dead cells, invading microorganisms, and white cells, and is the first defense mechanism of the body against localized infection.

rectum the lower part of the large intestine, which ends in the anus

rubber slang for a condom

salmonella bacteria which cause an intestinal infection and are sometimes sexually transmitted

salpingitis inflammation of the fallopian tubes, often caused by the spread of a sexual infection

scabies (*skay*-beez) a skin infection caused by a parasitic mite

scrotum the bag of thickened skin which holds the testicles and related structures

secondary infection   usually bacterial infection by streptococcus or staphylococcus of a site already infected (and therefore weakened) by another infection. Secondary infections are sometimes the result of scratching or other irritation where broken skin invites infection.

semen   (*see*-men) the milky fluid, made up of secretions from the testicles, prostate, and seminal vesicles, which is ejaculated at orgasm by a man. *One* component of semen (in a fertile male) is sperm.

seminal vesicles   a pair of small organs—one on either side of the prostate—which secrete one of the components of semen

shigellosis   a bacterial infection of the intestines caused by shigellae, and sometimes sexually transmitted

silent case   a subclinical, or asymptomatic, case of an infection. People with a silent case may be carriers of a disease without knowing it.

smegma   a thick, whitish, cheesy, smelly substance found under the foreskin of the penis or around the clitoris. It is an indication of lack of hygiene rather than infection.

speculum   an instrument to assist in the examination of a body cavity like the vagina

sperm   the male reproductive cell (technically spermatozoon) which fertilizes the female egg; *one* component of semen. A **spermicide** is a substance that kills sperm, used in contraceptive foams and jellies.

spirochete   a corkscrew-shaped bacterial organism, one type of which causes syphilis

sterile   not capable of producing offspring. Also said of an object free of organisms such as those that might cause infection.

strain   slang for gonorrhea, as in "have a strain"

stricture   a closing or narrowing of a passageway, often as a result of infection and subsequent scarring

syndrome   a group of symptoms which occur together and are characteristic of a particular disorder

syphilis   a bacterial sexual infection

tinea cruris   *see* jock itch

toxin   a poison which damages tissues by breaking them down and interfering with the ongoing life of a cell

trichomoniasis   a vaginal infection caused by protozoa called trichomonads

tubal pregnancy   an ectopic pregnancy—that is, one that develops in the fallopian tubes rather than in the uterus

ulcer   an open sore caused not by trauma but by infection, and characterized by diseased and disintegrating tissue

urethra the tube through which urine passes from the bladder and out through the urinary meatus. **Urethritis** is inflammation of the urethra.

urologist a specialist in problems of the urinary tract in both men and women, and of the reproductive tract in men

uterus the muscular, hollow, pear-shaped organ that receives the fertilized egg and protects it during its growth into a baby

vaginitis inflammation of the vagina

VD venereal disease: a contagious disease principally spread through sexual contact

VDRL a blood test for syphilis

venereal pertaining to sexual contact and/or pleasure

vulva the external female genitalia, including the labia (majora and minora), the clitoris (hood, shaft, and glans) and the vaginal introitus

warts, venereal a sexually communicated virus infection

wet-mount smear a sample of vaginal discharge prepared for examination. Wet-mounts by definition must be done on the spot; organisms may die if they dry out, and are then less easy to identify.

ABOUT THE AUTHORS

Stephani Cook has an M.A. in Family and Community Relations and has completed course work for a Ph.D. in Counseling Psychology at Teachers College, Columbia University. Her credentials in the area of sexuality include: work as a Counselor and Circulating Procedure Room Nurse at New York City's Center for Reproductive and Sexual Health; appointment to the Board of the Fertility Research Foundation in New York; teaching and consulting for International Planned Parenthood at the Margaret Sanger Clinic, New York City; Executive Director of HORIZONS in the Life Cycle, Inc., and a private practice in counseling, marital counseling, and sex therapy (certified as a sex therapist in 1973 by the Eastern Association of Sex Therapy and in 1979 by the American Association of Sex Educators, Counselors and Therapists). Ms. Cook also has taught and lectured and currently devotes full time to writing.

Richard Lumiere received his M.D. from Cornell University Medical College, served as an intern at the University of California at San Diego, and went on to do his residency in obstetrics and gynecology at New York's Lenox Hill and New York Hospitals. Dr. Lumiere has frequently given his time to free clinics in Georgetown and San Diego as well as in New York City, has served as attending gynecologist at the Fertility Research Foundation (New York City), and has spent two years in the Public Health Service in the Cancer Control Program. Among his numerous professional affiliations are the American Board of OB/GYN, American College of OB/GYN, Lenox Hill Hospital, and Doctors Hospital (New York City). Dr. Lumiere is the director of Women's Care Center in New York City and is a clinical instructor at New York Medical College. He has written frequently about women's health care for professional publications and maintains a private practice in New York City.